D1129994

AN INTRODUCTION TO WESTERN MEDICAL ACUPUNCTURE

Commissioning Editor: Karen Morley/Mary Law
Development Editor: Kerry McGechie
Project Manager: Elouise Ball
Designer: Stewart Larking
Illustration Manager: Bruce Hogarth
Illustrator: Adrian White and Cactus

AN INTRODUCTION TO WESTERN MEDICAL ACUPUNCTURE

EDITED BY

Adrian White
Editor, *Acupuncture in Medicine*
Clinical Research Fellow, Peninsula Medical School, Universities of Exeter and Plymouth, UK

Mike Cummings
Medical Director, British Medical Acupuncture Society
Honorary Clinical Specialist, University College London Hospitals
Senior Visiting Clinical Fellow, Bedfordshire & Hertfordshire Postgraduate Medical School

Jacqueline Filshie
Consultant in Anaesthesia and Pain Management, The Royal Marsden NHS Foundation Trust, Sutton, Surrey
Honorary Senior Lecturer, Institute of Cancer Research, Sutton, Surrey, UK

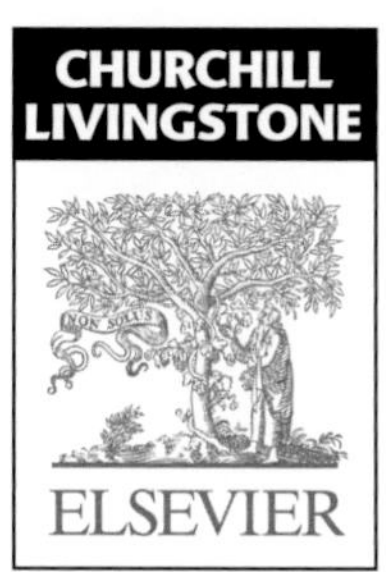

Hartness Library
Vermont Technical College
One Main St.
Randolph Center, VT 05061

Edinburgh London New York Oxford Philadelphia St Louis Sydney Toronto 2008

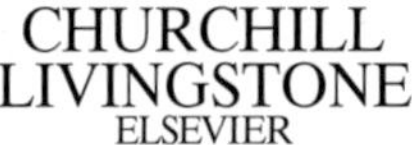

An imprint of Elsevier Limited

© 2008, Elsevier Limited. All rights reserved.

The rights of Adrian White, Mike Cummings and Jacqueline Filshie to be identified as authors of this work has been asserted by them in accordance with the Copyright, Designs and Patents Act 1988.

No part of this publication may be reproduced, stored in a retrieval system, or transmitted in any form or by any means, electronic, mechanical, photocopying, recording or otherwise, without the prior permission of the Publishers. Permissions may be sought directly from Elsevier's Health Sciences Rights Department, 1600 John F. Kennedy Boulevard, Suite 1800, Philadelphia, PA 19103-2899, USA: phone: (+1) 215 239 3804; fax: (+1) 215 239 3805; or, e-mail: *healthpermissions@elsevier.com*. You may also complete your request on-line via the Elsevier homepage (http://www.elsevier.com), by selecting 'Support and contact' and then 'Copyright and Permission'.

First published 2008

ISBN-13: 978-0-443-07177-5

British Library Cataloguing in Publication Data
A catalogue record for this book is available from the British Library

Library of Congress Cataloging in Publication Data
A catalog record for this book is available from the Library of Congress

Notice
Knowledge and best practice in this field are constantly changing. As new research and experience broaden our knowledge, changes in practice, treatment and drug therapy may become necessary or appropriate. Readers are advised to check the most current information provided (i) on procedures featured or (ii) by the manufacturer of each product to be administered, to verify the recommended dose or formula, the method and duration of administration, and contraindications. It is the responsibility of the practitioner, relying on their own experience and knowledge of the patient, to make diagnoses, to determine dosages and the best treatment for each individual patient, and to take all appropriate safety precautions. To the fullest extent of the law, neither the Publisher nor the Editors assumes any liability for any injury and/or damage to persons or property arising out or related to any use of the material contained in this book.

The Publisher

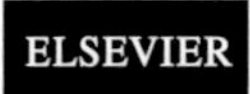
your source for books, journals and multimedia in the health sciences
www.elsevierhealth.com

Working together to grow libraries in developing countries
www.elsevier.com | www.bookaid.org | www.sabre.org
ELSEVIER BOOK AID International Sabre Foundation

The publisher's policy is to use **paper manufactured from sustainable forests**

Printed in China

FOREWORD

This excellent, authoritative and well-referenced book is in a class of its own because it is for the first time that the recently developed Western approach to acupuncture, based on the present-day neurophysiologic principles described in its pages, has been written about in such a lucid and wide-ranging manner.

All the various aspects of the subject are dealt with both comprehensively and cogently and from the information provided there can be no doubt that this particular form of acupuncture has a sound scientific basis and that its employment for certain well-defined disorders is becoming ever increasingly evidence-based.

It has been written by three eminent members of the British Medical Acupuncture Society, an organisation which over the 26 years since its inception has done so much to bring the principles and practice of scientifically-based acupuncture within the ambit of present-day orthodox medicine.

I therefore commend this book to all health professionals. The time has come when those who don't necessarily wish to use acupuncture themselves should nonetheless be aware of the indications for its employment so that they may be in a position to refer suitable patients where appropriate. Those who do wish to add it to their existing therapeutic skills will find this particular treatise to be an invaluable mine of information.

Peter Baldry MB; FRCP

PREFACE

There are numerous textbooks devoted to acupuncture, covering both theoretical and practical aspects of the therapy. The majority of books focus on traditional theory and practice, but this one takes quite a different view. It combines the latest ideas about the neurophysiological mechanisms of acupuncture with a practical approach that is directed largely by those mechanisms. Classical point locations and names are retained because they are useful and well known, but this book lays much greater emphasis on their segmental innervation than on any concepts of meridians.

Western medical acupuncture is used following an orthodox diagnosis and applies scientific principles, taking account of this diagnosis, to formulate a treatment to relieve symptoms. It is just one therapeutic method alongside others, and fits perfectly into the wider approach of the whole of Western medicine, which considers both the psychosocial and the physical wellbeing of the individual.

Thus, Western medicine that includes this form of acupuncture is one example of truly integrated medicine: a traditional therapy has been investigated, re-interpreted within a modern scientific context, and finally incorporated, where appropriate, within modern health care.

This book is a long-awaited companion to *Medical Acupuncture: a Western Scientific Approach.*

ACKNOWLEDGEMENTS

This book represents the ideas, knowledge and wisdom of many people, and the authors are grateful to everyone with whom they have had conversation, or whose articles they have read or lectures they have heard, and who have contributed in some way or other to this work, which tries to make sense of acupuncture in terms of Western science. They are literally too many to list here, and the references at the end of the book give some indication of the number and diversity of researchers who are engaged in the project of understanding acupuncture. We are also grateful for the help, patience and professionalism of Karen Morley and Kerry McGechie at Elsevier.

Despite the best intentions of all the above, we willingly accept responsibility for any errors or omissions.

CONTENTS

GLOSSARY

Term	Description
Please note: a list of classical meridians and their standard abbreviations appears in Tables 16.6 and 16.7 on page 218	
action potentials	A nerve's electrical response to stimulation; for example, by an acupuncture needle. The action potentials travel (or 'propagate') along the nerve fibre to the synapse (see below)
acupuncture point	Traditionally, a precise location where the needle should be inserted. Interpreted more loosely here
affective (component of pain)	The emotional aspect of pain, which is troubling or upsetting; 'the pain is awful'
afferent nerve	A nerve that brings information from the periphery towards the central nervous system – sensory nerve
analgesia	Analgesia strictly means complete removal of pain, but 'acupuncture analgesia' means pain reduction, often used in conjunction with anaesthesia from drugs
auricular acupuncture	Acupuncture in which needles are inserted into the external ear
autonomic nerves	Nerves responsible for controlling the body's functions that are not within conscious control
channel (=meridian)	Invisible lines on the surface of the body connecting acupuncture points. No physical structure to explain these channels has been found. In traditional Chinese medicine, channels are believed to be the route for the flow of '*qi*'
de qi	Chinese word for needle sensation, literally 'numbness, distension, heaviness and ache'; also tingling and spreading sensation
dermatome	The area of body surface innervated by a sensory nerve from a single spinal segment
dorsal horn	The part of the grey matter within the spinal segment where afferent nerves terminate

dry needling	A term sometimes used for acupuncture when needling is performed without a traditional Chinese approach
efferent nerve	A nerve that carries information away from the central nervous system, either motor or autonomic
electroacupuncture	Electrical stimulation applied through needles inserted in the usual way
extrasegmental	Not just limited to one spinal segment; used to describe one of the actions of acupuncture
laser 'acupuncture'	Low-energy laser applied to acupuncture points, without needles
limbic system	Collection of several centres within the brain which are closely involved in various emotional responses
major points	Acupuncture points that seem to have particularly strong generalized regulatory or stimulatory effects
meridian	See channel
moxa	Dried leaf of the plant *Artemisia vulgaris* used as a thermal stimulus. It is burnt either directly over the skin, or on or close to a needle. This treatment, *moxibustion,* was an integral part of traditional Chinese acupuncture treatment
myofascial trigger point	Small area of hyperirritability within a taut band of skeletal muscle that has particular characteristics
myotome	All the muscles innervated from a single spinal segment
NADA technique	Standardized form of auricular acupuncture for drop-in treatment centres for drug addicts, developed by the National Acupuncture Detoxification Association
neuropathic pain	Type of pain caused by malfunction of, or after injury to, the nervous system
neurotransmitter	Any chemical within the body that stimulates a nerve; and particularly one released by another nerve locally (neurotransmission)
nociception	The process of sensing a stimulus that could be harmful to the body; it may (or may not) give rise to the perception of pain
opioid peptides	A class of endogenous chemical transmitter within the CNS, whose overall effect is to modulate the perception of pain

pain	An unpleasant sensory and emotional experience, associated with actual or potential tissue damage, or described in terms of such damage
periosteal pecking	Stimulation of the periosteum with a needle
percutaneous electrical nerve stimulation	Effectively, the same treatment as electroacupuncture, though not using acupuncture points
placebo	An intervention that pretends to be a physical or chemical treatment, but works entirely psychologically; only ethical in the context of research
propagate	Correct term to describe the movement of action potentials along a nerve fibre
qi ('chi')	Often used to mean 'energy'. Originally represented nourishment and defence of the body (i.e. modern-day interpretation blood supply and immune function)
sclerotome	The area of bone innervated from a single spinal segment
sensitization	Excited state of the nervous system in which there is an exaggerated response to a stimulus. This can be peripheral or central
sensory stimulation	Treatments, including acupuncture, that involve stimulation of the sensory nerves. Practitioners who use this term are more likely to use electrical stimulation through pads or needles
sensory (component of pain)	The awareness of the pain in terms of site, nature and intensity: 'It hurts here' (see also 'affective' for psychological effect)
sensory stimulus	A physical modality that results in activation of sensory nerves
sham	= pretend. Usually in the context of a pretend treatment that is designed as a control procedure in a clinical trial
somatic	To do with the 'soma', which is basically the musculoskeletal parts of the body as distinct from the visceral parts
somatovisceral	The effect the body may have on the internal organs, by neural pathways
strong reactor	A patient who has much stronger adverse and beneficial reactions to acupuncture than most people
superficial needling	Needles enter the skin and superficial fascia, but do not penetrate deeper

synapse	The junction between two nerve cells, where the action potential in the first may transfer to the second, propagating the stimulus. The synapse is the crucial site where activity of the nervous system can be modified: local circumstances determine whether the effect of the incoming stimulus may be reduced, blocked or amplified
tender point	A location that causes pain when pressed; may or may not have the specific features of a myofascial trigger point
TENS	Transcutaneous electrical nerve stimulation, a technique of sensory stimulation through surface electrodes. Differs from acupuncture in important ways, especially in not (usually) having sustained or cumulative effects
traditional Chinese acupuncture	A mid-20th-century acupuncture approach that embraces various different models of acupuncture that evolved in different parts of China and at different historical periods. Part of traditional Chinese medicine (TCM)
viscerotome	All the organs innervated from a single spinal segment
viscerosomatic	The reflex effect that events in the internal organs have on the rest of the body, by neural pathways
Western medical acupuncture	An acupuncture approach that interprets acupuncture phenomena according to current understanding of the body's structure and function, and integrates acupuncture with Western medicine

CHAPTER

1

Introduction

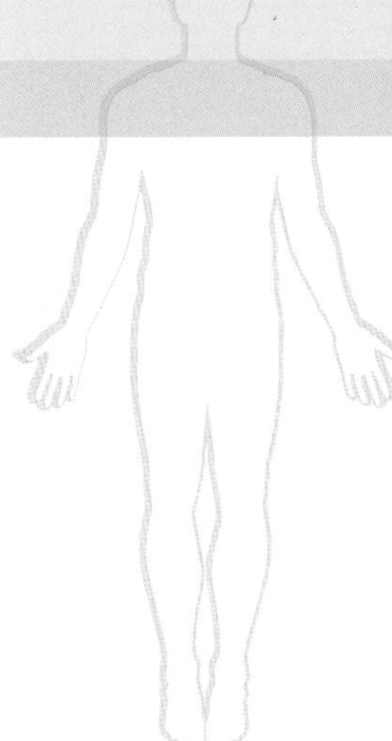

Contents

Treatment with acupuncture is a strange experience. Before lying down on the treatment couch, patients are likely to be asked to roll up their sleeves and take off their socks or stockings – even though they are not complaining of anything wrong with their hands and feet. The acupuncturist will probably poke and prod them in various parts of the body, and perhaps measure along the skin with his or her fingers, looking for a particular point to insert some special needles. The insertion itself is likely not to hurt at all, and certainly not like the sharp prick that you might expect – which is just as well, because the acupuncturist will go on inserting more needles, possibly as many as six or eight. The needles go either just into the skin or deeper into the muscle. Each needle is about 1 inch long (Plate 1), and is inserted up to about half way and then twiddled for 30 seconds or so. This produces an odd kind of ache, which is strange because the needles are solid – nothing is being injected and nothing is drawn out. Then the needles just rest there, or maybe they are attached to a battery-powered stimulator (Plate 2), which makes them gently tingle. The needles are left for about 10 to 20 minutes, before being simply taken out again. The patient then goes home, often feeling strangely relaxed for a few hours, even a bit sleepy. Then he or she may notice that the symptoms feel a bit better – though, just as likely, not after only one treatment. This strange performance is repeated once a week for a course of six or eight treatments, and in most cases the symptoms gradually disappear.

Patients who ask their acupuncturist what is going on, or who explore acupuncture on the internet or in a book, will probably be told something about acupuncture's origins in traditional Chinese medicine, and they will be told that the needles work by influencing something called '*qi*' energy, which flows round the body in structures called 'meridians'. These unusual ideas (which are not supported by any evidence, by the way) seem to match the strangeness of the treatment and so they tend to be accepted, even sometimes by people who recognize that they are completely foreign to our understanding of the way the body works. These explanations even seem to be accepted by some health professionals, and so it is easy for patients to accept them uncritically, thinking: 'The professionals should know, so why question them?'.

Readers of this book will discover a different approach: we take this strange therapy that has grown up over many centuries, and we try to re-interpret it in modern terms. We use a scientific viewpoint and apply the present-day understanding of the way the body works to explain what happens when those needles are inserted and manipulated. We hope to show that this medical approach can be used not only to explain what happens during acupuncture, but also as a guide to how to treat different conditions with needles. We hope this style of acupuncture will be more readily accepted in Western medicine, and so become more widely available to patients.

Let us summarize the position we take in this book:

- Acupuncture is a useful treatment that deserves a place alongside conventional drugs and surgery.
- There is a valid, modern approach to acupuncture that views it as a form of stimulation of nerve and muscle.
- We are not saying that our particular explanations are 'right' and traditional Chinese explanations are 'wrong'.
- We are not saying that science has provided all the answers – there are still plenty of gaps in our knowledge and understanding.
- The scientific approach is the best way to increase knowledge and understanding of acupuncture in the future, because it is self-critical by its very nature.

How can we be sure acupuncture is a valid therapy?

Acupuncture has often been dismissed without giving it much thought: after all, it is a really strange treatment and quite unlike any other treatment in the whole of medicine or surgery, and the usual explanations given for it are even odder. So we can understand when people think: 'It must be just suggestion'. We have our fair share of scepticism, but our experience of acupuncture convinces us that it is a real and valuable phenomenon. Here are just three lines of reasoning in support of that view:

1. Acupuncture is increasing in popularity, both among patients and among their doctors – some of whom have a reputation for being pretty hard-headed. The opinions of so many thousands of sensible people should not be dismissed too easily. In a UK survey in 1998, about 7% of the adult population reported that they had used acupuncture at some time in their life (Thomas et al 2001a). Acupuncture is increasingly used by general practitioners (GPs) themselves, or provided by other members of the primary healthcare team. It is the most popular of the complementary therapies (Thomas et al 2001b). Acupuncture is offered to patients in 84% of chronic pain clinics in the National Health Service (Woollam & Jackson 1998). In these pain clinics, competition for resources is intense and no treatment survives unless it works reasonably frequently. A similar picture emerges from other Western countries, and acupuncture

continues to be offered routinely in many countries in the East such as China, Korea and Vietnam, where it is usually available in parallel with mainstream Western-style medicine.

2. There is increasing evidence from clinical trials that acupuncture is not just a placebo. There are many difficulties in organizing really rigorous clinical trials of acupuncture, and not the least of these is what to use as the 'placebo' – after all, what else looks and feels like a needle, but is not a needle? However, there are now enough trials, and reviews of those trials, to be reasonably confident that acupuncture has real effects. Recent reviews have shown acupuncture to be better than placebo in treating three quite different kinds of problem: nausea and vomiting (Lee & Done 2004, Ezzo et al 2005), back pain (Manheimer et al 2005) and chronic knee pain (White et al 2007). There is plenty of positive evidence in other conditions and we summarize this later in the book.
3. Perhaps the most powerful argument in favour of acupuncture is the accumulated clinical experience that comes with watching patients being treated with acupuncture, and listening to their comments. The events that happen, both during and after treatment, are so distinctive and so unexpected that patients simply could not make them up. And they happen often enough, and are similar enough in completely different patients, to suggest that acupuncture needles have some quite definite and biological effects. Some of these events are listed in Box 1.1.

BOX 1.1

Phenomena that are characteristic of acupuncture treatment

- The needles produce sensations quite unlike anything else ever experienced.
- Pain relief occurs in three distinct patterns: sometimes immediately on removing the needles; sometimes the morning after treatment; and sometimes gradually accumulating over a course of several treatments.
- Needles in one part of the body treat another part: e.g. patients with migraine benefit from being needled in the foot.
- Patients spontaneously report feelings of improved wellbeing and deep sleep after treatment.
- Other minor symptoms (not known to the acupuncturist and quite incidental to the main problem being treated) are often improved by acupuncture, such as an irregular menstrual cycle, or a mild bowel disorder.
- Mild 'systemic' adverse events may occur after treatment, e.g. drowsiness, aggravation of symptoms, headache or nausea.
- Very occasionally, acupuncture produces a surprisingly strong impact on the nervous system (exceptionally, it may even cause a convulsion of some kind, or a loss of consciousness for a short time).

Why not simply accept the traditional explanations for acupuncture?

People tell us that, because the Chinese discovered acupuncture many centuries ago and are still using it, and because their explanations are so natural, beautiful and philosophical, they must be right. The same people tell us that our scientific approach is too limited to do justice to the subtleties of this ancient art. We are not convinced by this, and shall explain why briefly here (and in more detail later in the book).

Acupuncture developed over the course of 2000 years. During this period, theories about the world evolved and changed dramatically as people made new discoveries and achieved a fresh understanding of nature. With each new world view, the phenomena of acupuncture were explained in a different way, according to the new ideas. We are simply continuing this tradition.

Up till now, acupuncturists have been careful not to reject the earlier concepts but to add the new explanations on to the old. So, ancient Taoist concepts of Yin and Yang from Naturalism circa 300–400 BC, incorporated during the era of Han Confucianism circa 100 BC, mingle with ideas of disease due to possession by demons, theories of five fundamental universal elements and modern syndromes. There seems to have been a kind of respect for earlier models that made people hang on to the old ideas as some kind of insurance against losing valuable insights.

However, Western science has brought a whole fundamental change to the nature of our knowledge and understanding, and to keep hold of the old ideas while adding the new ones would be the equivalent of asking the reader to accept both that the world is round *and* that it is flat. That is not easy for the modern man.

We regard traditional Chinese acupuncture as a fascinating part of history of medicine, and we respect the ancient physicians, but their explanations are not meaningful today – at least, not to us. We shall illustrate this with just three examples of fundamental ideas in traditional Chinese acupuncture theory:

1. Traditional Chinese acupuncture involves the basic concept that acupuncture points exist on meridians and it is through the meridians that the needles achieve their effects. But nobody has shown any evidence for the physical existence of these meridians, so far. To get round this problem, the meridians are sometimes described as only an abstract concept: but it is difficult to accept how such an abstract concept can have the powerful physiological effects that we see in clinical practice.
2. Traditional Chinese acupuncture can offer an explanation for every individual's symptoms, and can offer a diagnosis for every condition in the medical dictionary. However, from what we know about the huge range of diseases that are part of medicine, it seems highly improbable that conditions as different as cancer, rheumatoid arthritis, pneumonia and heart disease can be explained by a single, all-embracing mechanism, let alone that they might all respond to treatment with acupuncture needles.

3. When it comes to the actual treatment with acupuncture, the points are selected on the basis that every acupuncture point has a specific function. For example, a point near the great toe 'clears Liver-Fire'. Even if we can understand the symptoms of 'Liver-Fire' as hot sensations and flushing of the skin, the idea that the underlying cause of these sensations can be corrected by needling a specific point in the foot is not meaningful, according to what we know of the anatomy and physiology of the body. This 'cause and effect' relationship seems to be the territory of science, not a traditional belief system, and explanations using the ideas that the needles stimulate nerves and release transmitters in the brain seem to us to be much more appropriate.

Readers will be forgiven for reaching the conclusion that, if they wanted to accept the theory of traditional Chinese acupuncture, they would have to 'suspend their disbelief'. It is time to reconsider acupuncture and its strange phenomena in ways that are credible to Western science.

Reassessing the phenomena of acupuncture

So this is the heart of our argument: acupuncture works, but not for the reasons usually stated. Acupuncture as a treatment is valid, but the traditional explanations do not apply in the modern world.

The aim of this book is to provide explanations that tie in with current understanding of structure, function and disease – plus a small amount of conjecture. We accept that these explanations are only provisional, and will be revised when new discoveries are made; but they provide a sound basis for treatment that is rational in the present circumstances. We believe this approach will make acupuncture accessible to many more patients.

The arrangement of the book aims to unfold our understanding of acupuncture methodically, starting with the underlying mechanisms of action (Section I), through evidence of safety and effectiveness (Section II), preparation for practice (Section III) and, finally, guidance for clinical practice (Section IV).

This book is intended for people who want to learn how to use acupuncture in their treatments. It must be seen as a supplement to practical 'hands on' training courses for healthcare practitioners and not as a substitute. Learning any practical therapy such as acupuncture must involve some observation and apprenticeship. It is not our aim to write a 'cookbook' of treatment recipes, but to help the reader understand the fundamental principles of acupuncture that can then be applied to any situation where it is appropriate.

Finally, a note about the use of literature references in this book: we do not aim to provide comprehensive scientific citation to support every factual statement we make: if we did that, the reference list would be longer than the text. We have tried to cite a reference to support all crucial steps in the arguments, and also tried to include all the major references that we believe will be useful to any reader who wishes to expand his or her knowledge on particular subjects.

An overview of Western medical acupuncture

CHAPTER 2

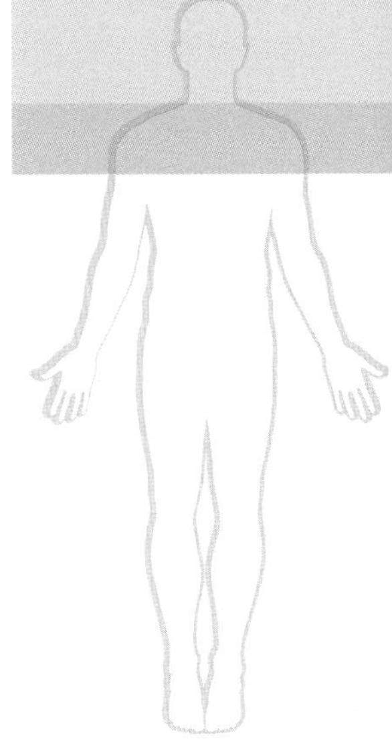

Contents

Introduction

This chapter gives a brief review of what we know about the physiological mechanisms of acupuncture and how they can provide a rational basis for treating patients. This is intended to be both a summary for the general reader and an introduction for the practitioner, so that the following chapters on mechanisms are more digestible. In this chapter, we avoid technical words where possible and we keep references to a minimum, to avoid distracting the reader.

To a casual observer Western medical acupuncture looks very similar to traditional Chinese acupuncture. Needles are inserted in various places in the body including often the hands and feet; they are agitated by hand and sometimes stimulated by electrical impulses and they are taken out again after a period of time; usually somewhere between 5 and 30 minutes.

However, there are considerable differences between the two approaches. A Western acupuncturist makes a medical diagnosis in the conventional way, uses needles to influence the physiology of the body according to the conventional (scientific) view, and regards the acupuncture as a conventional treatment along with drugs or surgery, or whatever else the patient requires. A traditional acupuncturist makes a diagnosis in terms of a disturbance in the body's 'balance', which needs to be corrected with needles.

Acupuncture in the West

Several British doctors discovered the benefits of acupuncture independently, over the last couple of hundred years. Early in the 19th century a London surgeon with the name of Churchill published two books on acupuncture describing how he treated patients with rheumatic pain by inserting needles into tender points (Baldry 2005a). A century later, the famous Canadian physician William Osler (1849–1919) discovered acupuncture and recommended inserting hat pins into tender points in the back muscles to treat lumbago. Neither of these eminent doctors used Chinese philosophy to explain acupuncture, but simply inserted needles into the painful points.

The modern history of Western medical acupuncture starts in the 1970s with Felix Mann, a medically qualified doctor who took the trouble to learn Chinese so that he could better understand the acupuncture that he had learned in both Europe and China. The conclusions he drew from his studies and from his clinical experience were quite heretical at the time: 'Meridians don't exist; points don't exist'. This liberated other acupuncturists to think the unthinkable and start to explore a rational approach to acupuncture.

About the same time, research had begun to provide the means to understand the mechanisms of acupuncture. Against the background of the gate control theory of pain (Melzack & Wall 1965), the discovery of the 'endorphins' (Hughes et al 1975) was a major advance, followed shortly afterwards by studies that showed that acupuncture released the endorphins (Han & Terenius 1982). This close association between acupuncture and the endorphins, now called 'endogenous opioid peptides', helped enormously to establish the credibility of acupuncture and this has been reinforced over time by discoveries of other mechanisms of action, as well as by positive clinical trials. Since the 1970s, Western medical acupuncture has gradually earned its place and become more widely accepted alongside conventional Western therapies in a modern health service.

Western medical acupuncture is based on a contemporary understanding of the body's mechanisms.

Five mechanisms for understanding Western medical acupuncture

Here we present five mechanisms (Fig. 2.1) that can go a long way towards explaining the phenomena of acupuncture, as they were outlined in the Introduction. Four of the mechanisms involve the nervous system and one involves the muscles. Each can be used for a different purpose, which is why anyone using Western medical acupuncture needs to understand the patient's condition in terms of its conventional diagnosis and pathology. The different mechanisms require slight variations in the treatment techniques, so these need to be tailored for the individual patient. In practice, there is considerable overlap between the mechanisms, and treatment often activates more than one mechanism.

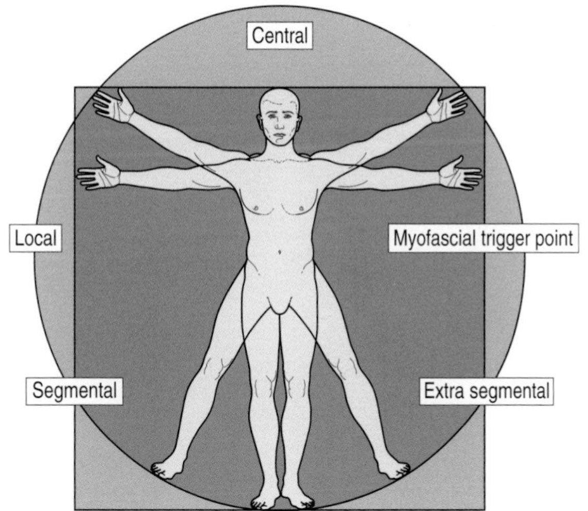

Figure 2.1 Five known mechanisms for the effects of acupuncture.

Local effects

Acupuncture produces many of its effects by stimulating nerve fibres in skin and muscle. These sensory nerves form a network in the layers of the skin. Needling one of these nerves sets off action potentials (see Glossary). The action potentials spread around the network locally, an effect that is known as an 'axon reflex'. Various substances are released as a result, particularly one called calcitonin gene-related peptide (CGRP). This causes the local blood vessels to dilate, so the local blood flow increases. This effect can often be seen in patients having acupuncture: the skin around the needles often flushes bright red with the increased blood flow (see Plate 3), and afterwards a small 'weal' can be seen under the skin (Plate 4). The blood flow is also increased in the deeper tissues, which encourages tissue healing, for example in some skin conditions or minor injuries. It may also improve the function of local glands, such as salivary glands.

Acupuncture promotes local healing.

Segmental analgesia

The action potentials also travel up the nerve directly to its particular segment in the spinal cord where they tend to depress the activity of the dorsal horn, reducing its response to painful stimuli. This is known as a 'segmental' effect, and is probably the main mechanism by which acupuncture relieves pain – the symptom it is most commonly used for. Acupuncture inhibits pain from any part of the body which sends nerves to that particular segment of the spinal

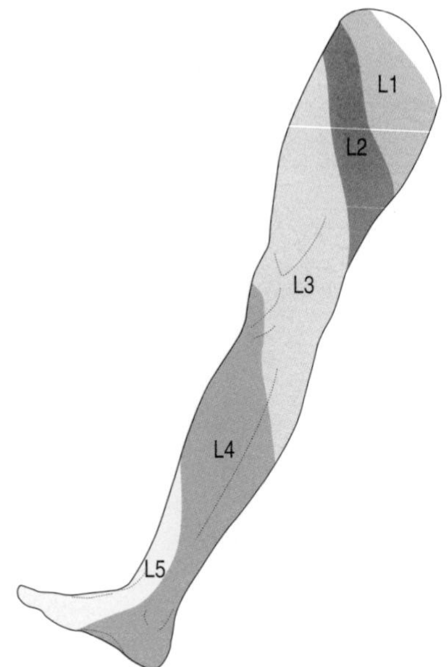

Figure 2.2 Schematic drawing of leg showing innervation of the skin by different spinal segments. An acupuncture needle reduces pain in the segment which it stimulates.

cord. For example, the nerves from a painful knee joint enter the same segment as the nerves from the muscles around it: so pain in the knee joint will be reduced by needles inserted in those muscles. Actually, because the connections of the nerves are not confined precisely to a single segment, the segmental effect of acupuncture spreads to the adjacent segments as well, as shown schematically in Figure 2.2.

Acupuncture reduces pain in the segment where the needles are inserted.

Extrasegmental analgesia

The action potentials produced by the acupuncture needle then travel on from the dorsal horn up to the brainstem. Here, they stimulate the body's own pain-suppressing mechanisms. If it is a surprise to learn that the body should have mechanisms to suppress pain, then remind yourself of occasions when you have injured yourself without really noticing, probably because you were concentrating hard on something else at the time – for example, while playing sport. Only when you relax after the match do you become aware of the pain (Melzack & Wall 1988). Clearly, the brain can inhibit pain, and it does this by descending nerves, which release some neurotransmitters at every segment of the spinal cord.

This is known as the 'extrasegmental' analgesic effect – because it is not restricted to a single segment. Acupuncture can activate the extrasegmental effect, and so have effects that extend to the whole body, well beyond the segment in which acupuncture is applied. The extrasegmental effect is not usually particularly powerful – not enough to suppress pain altogether – but every little helps.

Acupuncture reduces pain throughout the body.

The extrasegmental effect does not seem to depend on needling particular points, but more on the achievement of an adequate amount of stimulation.

Central regulatory effects

After reaching the midbrain, the action potentials go on to influence various other structures in the brain. One of these is the cerebral cortex, where the sensation of needling is registered. Other deeper structures are also stimulated, including the hypothalamus and limbic system. These are the sites of the various 'regulatory' effects of acupuncture. These changes in the brain are shown in the images in Plate 5, which we shall return to later in the book.

Acupuncture has general calming effects on many patients and improves their wellbeing. They become more cheerful and more motivated with a positive outlook on life, though this may be partly due to other factors in the therapeutic relationship. Patients may still feel the pain, but it bothers them less. Acupuncture also has other important central regulatory effects. It is well known for reducing nausea, for example in pregnant women. It may also influence the autonomic nervous system, and various hormones, such as the female hormones that control the menstrual cycle.

According to the Western approach, some of these effects of acupuncture depend more on the type of stimulation that is given than the precise location where it is given.

Acupuncture has a calming effect and improves wellbeing.

Myofascial trigger points

Everyone is familiar with the fact that broken bones, injured joints, strained ligaments and tendons are painful. But most people look on injuries to muscles as rather less serious and simply expect them to heal. In fact, when a muscle has been heavily overloaded or suddenly stretched – perhaps strained by an awkward posture at a desk, or perhaps by carrying something heavy – it can develop a small area of damage that can be slow to heal and cause persistent pain. Small 'knots' of tight muscle fibres form, known as a 'myofascial trigger point' (MTrP) (Fig. 2.3). These MTrPs are far from fully understood; they may be a protective mechanism to ensure the muscle rests while it heals, or they may simply be a malfunction of the process of healing in the muscle.

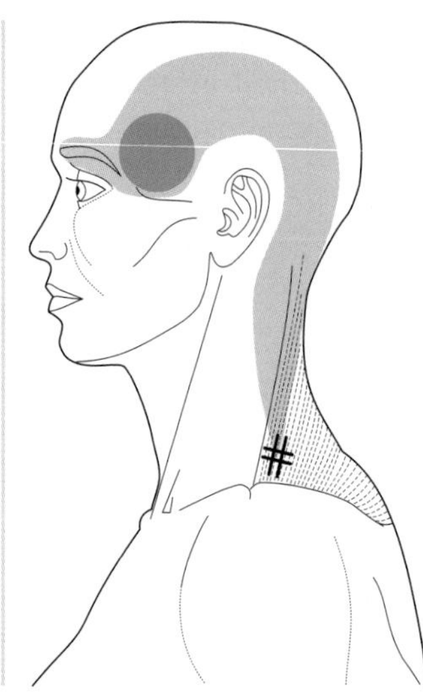

Figure 2.3 Myofascial trigger point in trapezius muscle causing pain in neck and head.

Myofascial trigger points are tender, but they are not just ordinary 'trigger points' and should be distinguished from the tenderness in fibromyalgia. Unfortunately, there is no blood test or X-ray examination that confirms the diagnosis, and we have to rely on careful examination to identify them. MTrPs can be distinguished by their typical features:

- A *taut band* can be felt running from one end of the muscle fibre to the other, with an acutely *tender spot*.
- The pain produced by pressure on the tender spot is recognized by the patient as his or her own pain.
- The pain is referred some distance away, in a predictable fashion (see Fig. 2.3). In fact, it is often possible to work backwards from the site of the pain and predict the site of the MTrP.
- The movement of the muscle is restricted by pain.

Various lines of evidence suggest that myofascial trigger points were recognized by the ancient Chinese physicians, and they could even have been among the earliest medical conditions to have been treated with needles.

Acupuncture inactivates myofascial trigger points.

Mechanisms not yet known

There are still large gaps in the understanding of neurophysiology of the human body, but two areas of current research should provide us with an even better understanding of acupuncture mechanisms within the next few years.

Firstly, the mechanisms of chronic pain are poorly understood, but current concepts that are being investigated and show promise include long-term changes in neurotransmitters and their receptors, and the changes to glial cells and the blood–brain barrier.

Secondly, imaging studies, particularly functional magnetic resonance imaging, are revealing the function of the brain and providing a new understanding of the actions of the deeper brain structures. These studies have already contributed to a greater understanding of acupuncture.

Additionally, more detail is being discovered about the local effects of acupuncture and some of these effects may not involve the nervous system directly. For example, evidence is already beginning to accumulate that acupuncture needles may have important effects on connective tissue.

The use of Western medical acupuncture

The term 'medical' acupuncture is not meant to imply that only doctors can use it and the words 'modern' or 'scientific' acupuncture would do equally well. They all convey the idea that this approach to acupuncture is based on the current understanding of the structure and function of the body. This is the fundamental difference from the traditional Chinese approach.

The essential features of treatment with Western medical acupuncture are that:

- conventional methods of medical history and examination are used, with clinical investigations if necessary, to establish a conventional diagnosis
- the functions that need to be influenced by acupuncture in a particular patient are decided upon
- the appropriate treatment is given, in a dose that is carefully tailored to the individual
- the treatment is repeated according to the patient's initial response and the changes they report over the subsequent few days.

Western medical acupuncture does not claim to treat every medical condition, nor every individual; acupuncturists need to know when it is appropriate, and when not appropriate, to use acupuncture.

Other interpretations of Western medical acupuncture

In this book we describe acupuncture treatment very much in terms of its mechanisms of action. We encourage the acupuncturist to plan a treatment in order to activate the mechanisms that will benefit the patient. This means that our approach is fairly and squarely 'evidence based' – and as a result it will be constantly modified and developed in the light of new research, and become acceptable in an evidence-based health service.

Other approaches to Western acupuncture by respected practitioners focus more on clinical examination and the experience of the practitioner. Mann rejects conventional points in most respects, and recommends minimal needling of a restricted number of points (Mann 1992). Campbell attaches great significance to the patient's reaction to both examination and needling, and uses 'acupuncture treatment areas' rather than traditional points (Campbell 2001). Both approaches rely heavily on learning by experience, but often the modern practitioner has rather little time to devote to the experimentation and careful observation that are needed to apply these approaches. Macdonald emphasizes the significance of the tender point (Macdonald 1982), and Baldry, another influential medical acupuncturist, emphasizes the treatment of trigger points after the pioneering work of Travell and Simons (Baldry 1993), and now recommends the routine use of superficial needling. Gunn has developed a particular application of acupuncture by concentrating on diagnosis and treatment of radiculopathy, considering this to be the fundamental cause of many cases of chronic pain. He treats the affected segments with deep needling of paravertebral points, a treatment called 'intramuscular stimulation' or IMS.

Other authorities have concentrated on a standardized form of stimulation, particularly electrical stimulation: in Sweden this treatment is called 'sensory stimulation' (Lundeberg 1999), and in the USA 'scientific acupuncture' (Ulett & Han 2002).

We recognize and draw on the experience and wisdom of all these experts, and encourage readers who want to explore all aspects of acupuncture to study their work.

The Western medical approach has been fostered in the UK by the British Medical Acupuncture Society, who aim to 'encourage the scientific understanding' of acupuncture by seeking evidence, rationalizing the treatment approach and distilling its essence on the teaching courses, which have been evolving since the Society's foundation in 1980.

Some schools of thought in acupuncture still cling to the traditional Chinese acupuncture ideology, but add Western physiological understanding to form a kind of hybrid version. Some of these also use the term 'medical acupuncture' (Helms 1998).

Milestones in Western medical acupuncture

Some of the main contributions to the re-evaluation of acupuncture in scientific terms are listed in Table 2.1, although there are countless other clinicians and scientists who have contributed to the critical thinking about acupuncture, and have helped to understand it.

TABLE 2.1

Milestones in the development of various aspects of Western medical acupuncture (developed from a table by Ulett 2002)

Date	Name(s)	Topic	Milestone
1952 on	Travell	Myofascial trigger pont (MTrP)	Exploration of myofascial origin of pain
1965	Melzack & Wall	Pain concepts	The gate control theory of pain
1973	Chiang et al	Basic research	Local anaesthetic blocks acupuncture effect
1975	Hughes et al	Basic research	Discovery of endogenous opioids
1970s on	Han; Pomeranz	Basic research	Acupuncture and neurotransmitter release
1970s on	Mann	Acupuncture concepts	Traditional concepts of acupuncture challenged radically
1977	Melzack	MTrP	Correlation between acupuncture points and myofascial trigger points
1977	Mayer	Basic research	Acupuncture analgesia reversed by naloxone
1980	Clement-Jones	Basic research	Opioid peptides rise in humans after acupuncture
1982	Han & Terenius	Basic research	Classic review article on neurotransmitter release by acupuncture
1980s	Lundeberg	Clinical research	Clinical trials on acupuncture for pain control
1980s	Dundee	Clinical research	Placebo controlled trials of acupuncture for nausea
1983	Travell & Simons	MTrP	Definitive manual of trigger point therapy published
1983	Hubbard	Basic research	Trigger points show electrical activity
1996	Vickers	Clinical research	First positive systematic review for acupuncture
1997	Gerwin	MTrP	Showed MTrP diagnosis to be reliable
1999	Simons	MTrP	Proposed mechanism for trigger points
1999	Lundeberg	Basic research	Demonstrated release of calcitonin gene-related peptide by acupuncture
2000	Hui	Basic research	Effects of acupuncture on the brain shown by magnetic resonance imaging
2005	Shah	Basic research	Microdialysis at myofascial trigger points demonstrates high levels of substances that sensitize afferent nerves
2005	Pariente	Basic research	Real needle activates ipsilateral insula, placebo needle does not

Further reading

Baldry P 2005 Acupuncture, trigger points and musculoskeletal pain. Churchill Livingstone, Edinburgh

A thorough and detailed textbook that contains valuable information about the development of acupuncture, modern theory of mechanisms of acupuncture, extensive acupuncture diagrams of myofascial trigger points.

Campbell A 2001 Acupuncture in practice: beyond points and meridians. Butterworth-Heinemann, Oxford

A highly readable individual account of medical acupuncture introducing the idea of an Acupuncture Treatment Area, to replace traditional points.

Mann F 1992 Reinventing acupuncture: a new concept of ancient medicine. Butterworth-Heinemann, Oxford

A personal record by an author who has been at the forefront of Western medical acupuncture, with excellent illustrations as part of an extensive guide to treatment.

CHAPTER

3

Neurological mechanisms I: local effects

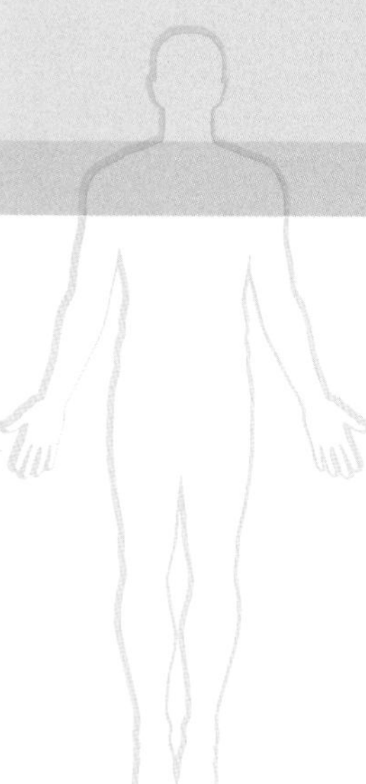

Contents

After reading this chapter you should be able to:

- name the type of nerve fibre that is stimulated by acupuncture
- name two neuropeptides released locally by acupuncture.

Introduction

Different types of acupuncture treatment have developed for different purposes. The simplest form is to insert one or a few needles into skin or muscle where you want to have the effect – around an area of inflamed or painful skin, for example. This is *local* treatment, and is the subject of this chapter.

We shall first describe the local organization of the sensory nerves, then the physiology of needling, then the way this information can be used to guide clinical practice. We shall then be in a position to discuss the rational basis for needling techniques.

We have the Chinese to thank for the first scientific investigations of acupuncture and the discovery that acupuncture operates through the nervous system. One crucial experiment in the early days of acupuncture research showed that acupuncture needles had no effect if they were inserted into an area that had been anaesthetized by injection of a local anaesthetic (Chiang et al 1973). Another trial showed that acupuncture generates nerve action potentials that can be detected in the nerve trunks leading away from the area being treated (Wang et al 1985). This pioneering work leaves us in no doubt that acupuncture stimulates nerves.

Sensory nerves

The main sensory nerves that are found in skin and muscle are shown in Table 3.1. The evidence strongly suggests that the clinical effects of acupuncture mainly involve the small myelinated nerve fibres: in the skin, these are the Aδ fibres, and in the muscle they are the type II/III nerves in muscle. The term 'Aδ' is more catchy than 'type II/III' so, simply for convenience, we shall refer to these small myelinated fibres as 'Aδ' fibres throughout this book, even though most acupuncture probably stimulates the type II/III fibres in muscle. The free nerve endings of these small myelinated fibres are organized in broad networks, as we show schematically in Figure 3.1.

Acupuncture stimulates small myelinated (called Aδ) fibres in skin and muscle.

Physiology of local acupuncture

Needle sensation: *de qi*

Acupuncture needles may produce needle sensation that the Chinese called *de qi*. This sensation was traditionally described as having four components (Lu & Needham 1980):

1. Numbness
2. Distension/extension/fullness
3. Heaviness
4. Sour ache 'like a feeling of muscular fatigue'.

TABLE 3.1

Classification of the main sensory nerve fibres in skin and muscle

Fibre type	In skin	In muscle	Ending	Sensation
Large myelinated	–	I	Muscle spindle – primary	None
Large myelinated	Aβ	II	Encapsulated and free endings	Light touch, pressure, vibration
Medium myelinated	Aγ	II	Muscle spindle – secondary, encapsulated endings	Numbness
Small myelinated	Aδ	III	Free endings	Deep pressure, heaviness in muscle, pinprick in skin, cold
Small unmyelinated	C	IV	Free endings	Soreness, aching, itch, heat; calmness[a]

[a]Stimulation of some small unmyelinated fibres induces calmness, with little cortical awareness.

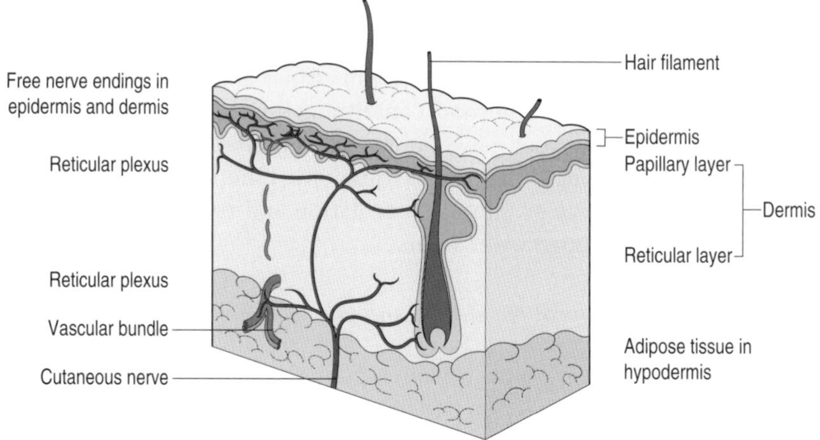

Figure 3.1 Schematic illustration of the arrangement of sensory nerves in the skin. Stimulating any part of the nerve affects the whole local network.

Patients also describe the sensations of pressure, tingling, warmth or cold, and the spreading or radiation of sensations (Hui et al 2000, Vincent et al 1989). These *de qi* sensations can usually be identified separately from the sensations of simply being pricked with a needle – sharpness or pain. Patients may feel either, or both, but it is the *de qi* sensation that is peculiar to acupuncture, and a mark that the nerve has been successfully stimulated.

Nerve conduction studies have shown that the onset of *de qi* is accompanied by action potentials that travel at the speed, and have the waveform appearance, typical of stimulation of Aδ fibres (Wang et al 1985). In addition, the aching, heavy sensation of *de qi* is comparable to the deep muscle ache after exercise (Andersson & Lundeberg 1995) that arises from stimulation of the free endings of type II/III fibres.

The arrival of the sensation *de qi* was interpreted in TCM as indicating 'the gathering of the *qi*', the event that is necessary in producing a response. This is not so very far away from our interpretation according to current Western medical concepts – *de qi* is taken as an indication that the right nerves are being stimulated.

Rather confusingly, the term *de qi* is also used to describe the sensation the practitioner becomes aware of when the tissues seem to grab the acupuncture needle as it is rotated to and fro in the point, though this is less likely when using modern highly polished needles.

Local neuropeptide release

The acupuncture needle stimulates the free nerve endings to produce action potentials that spread locally around the meshwork or 'reticulum' of nerves (see Fig. 3.1) in what is known as an *axon reflex*. This stimulates the release of several neuropeptides that cause vasodilation and an increase in local blood flow.

One particular neuropeptide that has been studied in relation to acupuncture is calcitonin gene-related peptide (CGRP) (Dawidson et al 1998); others include nerve growth factor (NGF), vasointestinal active peptide (VIP) and neuropeptide Y. CGRP is a normal constituent of the sensory nerve, being synthesized in the dorsal root ganglion and transported to the periphery (i.e. in the opposite direction to nerve transmission). One of its functions in the periphery is nutritional: it promotes vasodilation and formation of new blood vessels, so facilitating repair after injury.

Acupuncture improves local blood flow and promotes healing.

There is often some redness of the skin around the acupuncture needle during or after treatment, particularly on the trunk; a sign of the release of vasoactive neuropeptides including CGRP and histamine. Sometimes fluid extravasation also occurs and a weal can be seen, which is similar to that seen as a result of the release of histamine (Plate 4). The patient may feel itchiness.

Experiments have shown that the blood flow in the skin and muscle of healthy volunteers increases as soon as a needle is inserted into the skin, and increases further when the needle is advanced into the underlying muscle, and increases still further when the needle is stimulated and *de qi* elicited (Sandberg et al 2003).

The local release of neuropeptides by acupuncture can influence other structures in the vicinity. For example, acupuncture points in the face can affect the activity of salivary glands. Patients with dry mouth due to post-irradiation xerostomia recorded an increase in saliva production after acupuncture at local points around the salivary glands (Blom et al 1993).

Other possible local mechanisms

Direct stimulation of nerve endings may not be the whole story, and one research group in particular are investigating the changes to the connective tissue caused by the mechanical stimulation through rotation of an acupuncture needle, and suggest mechanical transduction could be a significant mechanism for acupuncture (Langevin et al 2006).

Clinical application

For this most basic form of acupuncture, simply insert a few needles close to the area where an increase in circulation would be beneficial, for example round a soft-tissue injury that is slow to heal or close to an underactive salivary gland. The needles have to be inserted into healthy skin with an intact nerve supply. Local acupuncture is also used for local skin lesions and areas where the circulation is compromised. It may be convenient to surround the area with a ring of needles about 2.5 cm apart (since the axon reflex covers a 25 mm radius). This treatment was known picturesquely by the Chinese as 'fencing in the dragon' (see Fig. 3.2).

Only insert needles into healthy skin with intact nerves.

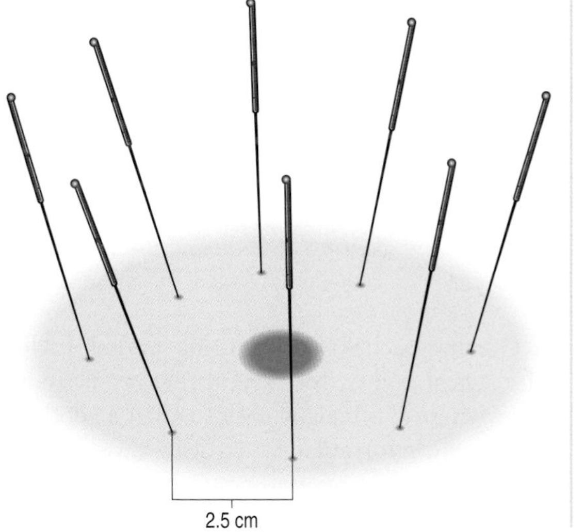

Figure 3.2 Needles surrounding a local skin lesion, known as 'fencing in the dragon'.

It has been suggested that the axon reflexes can operate over much longer distances and that this may turn out to explain some of the remote effects of acupuncture treatment that are otherwise difficult to explain (Carlsson 2002).

We can now set out some principles, based on the known physiology of acupuncture, to answer the two basic questions every acupuncturist needs to know, and which will occupy us throughout this book: Where should the needle be placed and how should it be stimulated?. There is no single answer to these questions; it all depends on what mechanism needs to be activated for each clinical situation.

Where to place the needle?

Local effects can be obtained by needling almost anywhere, but there also exist throughout the body certain sites that have come to be regarded as specially effective, the classical 'acupuncture points'.

Acupuncture points

Acupuncture points are a rather obvious and well-known feature of acupuncture. They are usually thought of as the recognized sites that are described in books and on anatomical charts. According to authoritative sources there are 361 points, mostly arranged in 'meridians', which can be seen on charts (The Academy of Traditional Chinese Medicine 1975). This all gives the impression that acupuncture points are precise, fixed locations that everybody agrees on, but this is actually far from true. Acupuncture students who have just been trained in college do not agree where the points are. Even the experienced lecturers in acupuncture who taught one of the authors at a recognized college disagreed over the precise location of some points. There is no objective test for points, such as temperature change or electrical skin resistance. Considerable research into acupuncture points has basically shown no particular identifying features. There is certainly no unique receptor or other structure for the acupuncture needle to activate.

The precise location of 'acupuncture points' is not as reliable as the experts suggest.

Our approach is this. We think it is helpful for acupuncturists to learn a number of classical points, for several reasons: acupuncture points are convenient locations where it is usually easy to elicit a good *de qi* sensation; some points appear repeatedly in formulae for treating a wide variety of conditions, probably because they have rather general, neurological effects – we call these the 'major' points; and other points are useful because they are used to treat common conditions. In addition, the names of the acupuncture points provide a reasonably consistent way to report where you inserted the needle, both for keeping a record and for reporting in papers or discussing with other practitioners.

However, we do not think Western medical acupuncturists need to worry too much about the precise location of these points to the nearest millimetre. Learn the rough location then use the finger tip as a guide to where to insert the needle. Experienced practitioners of Western medical acupuncture generally find they use a limited number of classical points, the major points, over and over again, as well as many other unnamed points that, for one reason or another – usually because they are tender – seem right for their patients.

A small number of major points can be used in classical formulae for treating many different conditions.

Numbering system of acupuncture points

We shall continue to use the classical numbering for acupuncture points simply because there is no other accepted scheme. On the chart, each point lies on a 'meridian' (which, as you imagine, is not a physical structure, as we discuss later) and this is usually named after an organ of the body, such as Liver or Gall Bladder. All the points on each meridian are numbered in sequence, but, inconveniently, the meridians are not all numbered in the same direction! So the standard abbreviation for a point consists of two capital letters, e.g. LU, LI, ST, and a number. The letters stand for Lung, Large Intestine and Stomach respectively, so typical points are labelled LU7, LI4, ST36 (see Tables 16.6 and 16.7 on p. 218 for full list). This is the nomenclature that has been established by international convention and we shall use throughout this book. Unfortunately, other nomenclature systems still survive.

The names of the meridians have nothing to do with the actual internal organ, as far as is known. In written text, it is easy to distinguish between

'Liver' as the meridian and 'liver' as the organ. But in talking to patients, they are naturally very interested when they hear you say you are going to treat 'Liver 3' or 'Gall Bladder 34', for example. They may even tend to assume there is something wrong with their actual liver or gall bladder and need an explanation.

Annoyingly, some points that are quite useful today were only introduced long after the original charts were defined, and so had to be labelled as 'Extra points'. These are usually referred to by their Pinyin names, without any numbers. We shall come across an example of this with two useful points on the face (*Yintang* and *Taiyang*), as well as a whole line of points close to the thoracic and lumbar spine, the *Huatuojiaji* (pronounced 'hwa-two-oh-cha-chi') points.

Even more annoyingly, there are different versions of the sequence of numbers in one meridian, Bladder (BL). One system numbers down to the knee before returning to the top of the back and descending again; the other system reaches the sacrum then turns back up before descending again. Both systems use the same numbering below the knee.

The classical numbering for acupuncture points is a convenient convention.

Needle stimulation: the acupuncture 'dose'

The overall amount of stimulation you give the patient may be more significant than the exact location where it is given. This is the 'dose' of acupuncture and it depends on several factors, like the number of points treated at a time, the depth of needling and the strength of stimulation. Because there has been so little research into these different factors, we are still unsure about the contribution each of them makes to the total dose of a treatment. However, empirically, it is important to be able to vary the dose to suit the patient and the condition, and we shall repeatedly return to this subject throughout the book. Here we shall summarize the main factors and then the way they can be combined into what we might regard as a 'standard' acupuncture treatment.

Number of needles

The appropriate dose of acupuncture may require insertion of a single needle or up to about 20. However, as a general rule, we advise only using up to about four or six needles for the initial treatment, in order to observe the response. This is because some patients seem very sensitive to acupuncture.

Thickness of needles

Clinical experience seems to support the intuitive concept that thicker needles (larger diameter of the shaft) provide stronger stimulation, which may simply be due to the fact that they are stiffer and exert more pressure when they are manipulated.

Depth of insertion

We shall consider needling into muscle as the standard technique for the purposes of this book; even though many acupuncturists only needle the skin and subcutaneous tissues. For example, Japanese acupuncturists use superficial needling for many conditions and some medical acupuncturists generally prefer to use superficial needling for myofascial trigger points (Baldry 2005b, Macdonald 1982). We discuss this again later in the book. It may be less easy to achieve the full-blown *de qi* phenomenon with superficial needling, though there is no doubt that some sensations can occur.

Needle manipulation to elicit *de qi*

The *de qi* sensation may occur spontaneously after the needle has been inserted, but usually the acupuncturist needs to elicit it actively by stimulating the needle. It is generally enough to rotate the needle between finger and thumb, but it may be necessary to include an up-and-down movement as well, sometimes called sparrow-pecking (Fig. 3.3). In this way, the needle reaches enough nerves to generate *de qi*. Quite often, the acupuncturist will feel a tightening of the tissues at about the same time as the patient experiences *de qi*.

Clinical experience suggests that patients who feel *de qi* are more likely to respond to the treatment.

One thing is clear: there is no need to treat so vigorously that C fibres are stimulated. Acupuncture can be effective without being unpleasant or aversive. It has to be admitted that some Chinese acupuncturists treat their patients strongly, but until there is clear evidence that this is necessary, and for what patients and what conditions, acupuncturists should avoid painful stimulation. As we discuss later, if a patient needs stronger stimulation then it is much preferable to use electrical stimulation than to manipulate the needles very forcefully.

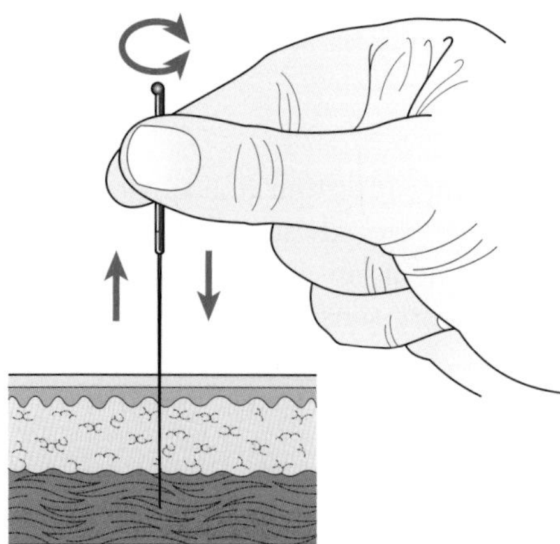

Figure 3.3 Two methods of manipulating a needle to elicit *de qi*.

Acupuncture does not need to be painful.

Needle retention time

For most conditions, the needle should be left in place for 10 to 20 minutes, but this can be varied according to the patient's response. Some acupuncturists find they can obtain results with as little as 30 seconds' needling. At the other extreme, needles can be left for 1 hour or more, for example to reduce pain in the postoperative period. For many patients, there is probably not much difference between the effects of retaining the needles for a few minutes compared with half an hour.

Standard treatment dose

A standard treatment is described in Table 3.2. Each of the variables can be adjusted to take account of the patient's medical condition, general physical condition, immediate responses during needling and (in subsequent treatments) the changes reported in the hours and days following needling.

Care and skill are needed to give the right dose of acupuncture.

Summary

This chapter describes the mechanisms of acupuncture when used to treat local conditions. Acupuncture achieves many of its actions by stimulating Aδ fibres, particularly in muscle. This produces a dull aching sensation known as *de qi*.

Acupuncture stimulates an axon reflex in the terminal network of Aδ fibres, which leads to local release of several substances. Calcitonin gene-

TABLE 3.2

Standard dose of acupuncture for local treatment

Variable	Typical for standard treatment
Points	2.5 cm intervals around area
Number of needles	Between 1 and about 8
Depth of insertion	Superficial for skin lesions
Needle stimulation	Manual stimulation, once after insertion
Response elicited	*de qi*
Needle retention time	10 minutes

related peptide (CGRP) is the best studied, and is known to improve blood flow locally and thus promote healing. This effect can be used to treat local skin lesions, or to improve the function of glands.

Acupuncture treatment involves decisions on where to insert the needle and what dose to give. Acupuncture points are not precisely agreed locations, but they are usually good places to elicit *de qi,* and using them can save time in practice. The dose, or strength of stimulation, depends on the number of needles, the depth of insertion, manipulation to elicit *de qi* and the needle retention time. For most conditions it is probably more important to give the right dose of acupuncture stimulation than to select exactly the right point.

CHAPTER

4

Neurological mechanisms II: segmental analgesia

Contents

After reading this chapter you should be able to:

- summarize the effect of acupuncture in the dorsal horn
- state the principle of segmental analgesia
- state three sites where you might choose points to treat bladder dysfunction, and give the reasons.

Introduction

The last chapter discussed the simplest of all treatments, local needling. This chapter deals with the next step, the treatment of an area such as a painful joint. This typically involves inserting a few needles around the joint, and perhaps one or two more further along the limb, stimulating them by twirling them between the fingers for about 1 minute, and then leaving them in position for at least 10 minutes. This is called *segmental* treatment because it operates at the level of the spinal segment.

This chapter concentrates on the mechanism of acupuncture in the spinal cord, particularly the dorsal horn. Firstly, it deals with acupuncture and the nerves from *somatic* (basically, musculoskeletal) structures and then it describes the effects of acupuncture on the autonomic nerves that innervate the *viscera* or internal organs. The mechanisms are basically similar, but the organisation of the autonomic system means that the approach with acupuncture treatment needs to be slightly modified.

In the following chapter, we reproduce a diagram that summarizes the mechanisms of action of acupuncture analgesia, as well as transcutaneous electrical nerve stimulation (TENS), and dorsal column stimulation analgesia, in different sites in the nervous system. This detailed diagram is intended as a reference source for the reader when studying both this chapter and the subsequent one, which discusses the mechanisms of acupuncture higher up in the nervous system, i.e. in the brainstem and the brain itself.

Somatic afferents: anatomy and physiology

Afferent nerve pathways: small unmyelinated and myelinated nerves

The afferent nerves enter the dorsal horn of the spinal cord. It is here that we see the first differences in the pathways of the nerves concerned with pain (the small unmyelinated or C fibres) and those concerned with acupuncture, the Aδ fibres, as illustrated in Figure 4.1. Note that we use the term 'Aδ' to include both the true Aδ fibres in skin and the type II/III fibres in muscle, which acupuncture needles stimulate.

Both types of fibre project onto some form of *transmission* cell in the dorsal horn – the unmyelinated fibres through a short chain of substantia

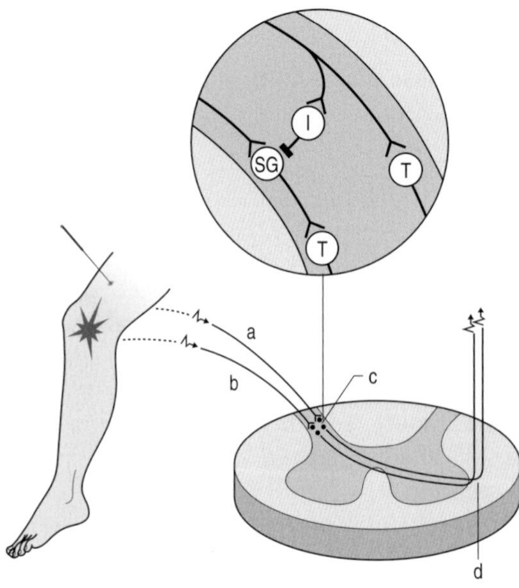

Figure 4.1 Section of spinal cord, showing projections of (a) acupuncture stimulus (myelinated nerve) and (b) noxious stimulus (unmyelinated nerve) to the dorsal horn (c). Pathway continues up anterolateral tract (d). Enlarged section of C shows how acupuncture stimulus can depress the response of substantia gelatinosa cell, leading to inhibition of pain. Key: SG = substantia gelatinosa cell; T = transmission cell; I = intermediate cell; + = facilitation; – = inhibition.

gelatinosa (SG) cells, and the myelinated fibres directly. The myelinated fibres also make collateral connections to small cells called *intermediate* cells, which have one particularly important property, crucial for acupuncture – they inhibit the activity of the SG cells.

The axons from the transmission cells cross to the opposite side of the spinal cord (to the anterolateral tract, also called the spinothalamic tract) and project up to the reticular formation in the *brainstem*, as shown in Figure 4.2. This is where the extrasegmental effects of acupuncture originate, as described in the next chapter.

From the brainstem, many fibres then project onto cells in the *midbrain* and *thalamus* – which are closely involved in the central regulatory effects of acupuncture, as described in Chapter 6.

From the thalamus, axons project to both:

- The somatosensory cortex, which registers the *sensory* aspect of pain – its location, duration and severity
- The *limbic system*, which deals with the unconscious processing of pain. This has various component parts, one of the most important being the *anterior cingulate cortex* (ACC), which registers the *affective* component of pain – its unpleasantness or psychological impact.

The above description is somewhat simplified, but adequate for our purposes. It is important to recognize that both the ascending pathways also make a large number of cross-connections to other centres throughout the central nervous system.

The perception of pain

According to the historic theory of pain perception, originally developed by Sherington, there was a fixed relationship between the severity of an

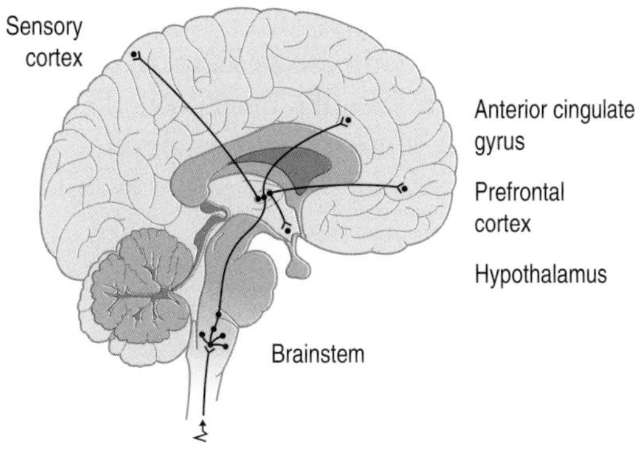

Figure 4.2 Schematic view of the central nervous system (sagittal section) showing the central pathways of the sensory afferents. They project first to the brainstem, where they activate descending inhibitory pain control; then they project onward to the thalamus, from where pathways travel both to the sensory cortex and to various parts of the limbic system (including the anterior cingulate cortex, prefrontal cortex, hypothalamus and other centres). Different stimuli acting on Aδ and C fibres activate the various target regions of the brain differentially.

injury and the resulting pain: the theory held that, if the injury was sufficient to stimulate the pain fibres, then the cortex of the brain would automatically be activated and the person would feel pain in proportion to the trauma.

It has become clear that the relationship between the degree of the trauma and the severity of the pain is far from fixed, and depends very much on the state of the nervous system at the time. The perception of pain from a particular injury can be reduced or increased:

- Inhibition: sometimes even major injury to the tissues does not cause pain; for example, in people who are severely injured in battle. This ability of the body to suppress pain is something we are interested in with acupuncture.
- Sensitization: sometimes a minor stimulus can cause severe pain because the nervous system responds in an exaggerated way; this is discussed in Chapter 6.

We now recognize that a traumatic stimulus that we might think of as 'painful' might not actually cause the sensation of pain. Therefore, it is more accurate to refer to the stimulus as 'noxious' rather than 'painful'. What was formerly called the pain pathway is now the nociceptive pathway, i.e. able to perceive noxious stimuli.

A noxious stimulus is one that potentially damages tissue; whether it registers as painful or not depends on the status of the nervous system.

Physiology of segmental acupuncture

Acupuncture needles stimulate small myelinated ('Aδ') nerves in muscle and skin; these activate the small intermediate cells in the dorsal horn, by way of collateral terminals. The intermediate cells release the neuromodulator *enkephalin*, which blocks the transmission of pain in the substantia gelatinosa cells, part of the nociceptive pathway (from the unmyelinated C fibres). The effect of enkephalin can be detected as a generalized depression of activity of the dorsal horn (Sandkuhler 2000). The effect is known as 'segmental analgesia', and takes some minutes to develop, but then outlasts the duration of the acupuncture stimulation, possibly even lasting several days.

Segmental analgesia – inhibition of the nociceptive pathway at approximately the same spinal level in the dorsal horn.

Note, for comparison, that segmental analgesia can also be produced by vibration and an electrical equivalent, transcutaneous electrical nerve stimulation (TENS). These stimulate the large myelinated (Aβ) fibres, which enter the dorsal column of the spinal cord. Like the Aδ fibres, the Aβ fibres also have collaterals that inhibit the transmission of nociceptive stimuli – but in this case, by the release of γ-aminobutyric acid (GABA), rather than met-enkephalin. This is the basis of the gate control theory of Melzack and Wall as originally described (Melzack & Wall 1965).

Clinical application of segmental analgesia

Segmental analgesia with acupuncture can be achieved simply by stimulating nerves in the same spinal segment as the origin of the pain.

Consider a patient with chronic knee pain from osteoarthritis. The noxious stimuli from the pain sensitive areas (probably the synovium, attachments of the joint capsule and subchondral bone) travel in the small unmyelinated C fibres into the dorsal horn mainly at the levels L3/L4 and L5/S1. (This follows the general rule: joints are innervated by the same segments that supply the muscles that act on them.) Acupuncture needles placed in vastus medialis (L2–4) and tibialis anterior (L4–5) will cover the appropriate segments nicely, and it is no coincidence that there are well-known traditional acupuncture points in both these muscles. They are called SP10 (Spleen 10) and ST36 (Stomach 36) respectively.

The spinal segment that supplies a joint also supplies the muscles that act on it.

Needling those muscles suppresses pain in the joint.

Sometimes the relevant segmental points can be some distance from the problem, but often they are very close. What about their local effect, as we described in the last chapter? A needle near to an area of pathology will both have local effects and produce segmental analgesia – all the more reason to insert it there.

Local needles can have local and segmental effects.

In practice, some analgesia can be also obtained by stimulating nerves in adjacent segments, since each afferent nerve actually influences more than one segment in the spinal cord. Therefore, adding more needles in the adjacent segments is the best way to increase the stimulation to the segment and increase the pain relief. For example, other classical acupuncture points around the knee are innervated by the same or adjacent spinal segments, and are often included in the treatment of knee pain. These points are often on the same meridians as the points around the knee, which leads to the traditional Chinese acupuncture concept of treatment using 'points in a line' – meaning distal points on the meridian that crosses the joint.

Needles need to be retained long enough to release enkephalin from the intermediate cells. A typical standard dose of acupuncture for segmental analgesia is shown in Table 4.1.

Segmental analgesia can have knock-on effects that may lead to some improvement in the condition, not just pain relief. The analgesia will reverse any increased muscle tone, so encouraging mobilization, which in turn

TABLE 4.1

Standard dose of acupuncture for segmental treatment

Variable	Typical for standard treatment
Points	Classical or tender points in same segment
Number of needles	Typically three to six
Depth of insertion	Intramuscular
Needle stimulation	Manual stimulation, possibly electroacupuncture
Response elicited	*de qi*
Needle retention time	10–20 minutes

improves blood flow and healing. Acupuncture analgesia may also improve the situation by reducing pain-related neurogenic inflammation.

The analgesia gradually wears off over several days, but can be reinforced by repeating the acupuncture and the benefits accumulate over a course of treatment. In this way, even chronic pain can respond to acupuncture.

Segmental analgesia may reduce any increased muscle tone, improving mobility and pain relief.

Electroacupuncture

Another way to increase the strength of stimulation is to use *electroacupuncture* (EA) – which involves running a small electrical current through the needles. As it is not essential to know about EA when starting to practise acupuncture, and since it involves aspects of a technical nature, we shall not introduce it as a treatment technique in these early theoretical chapters. It is described in detail in the chapter on effective needling techniques (Chapter 12).

Segmental acupuncture for visceral conditions

We have just seen that acupuncture reduces the perception of pain by acting on nerves in musculoskeletal structures. These are somatic afferents, but the effect of acupuncture is not limited to somatic afferents, but also reduces the response of the dorsal horn to any nociceptive information arriving there. So acupuncture can inhibit nociceptive stimuli from visceral structures such as the gut, bladder and uterus. In considering how to approach treating visceral problems with acupuncture, we have to modify our thinking about segmental analgesia in two ways:

1. The problem of needle location: whereas it is easy to place a needle close to a painful joint, it is not easy to place it close to an internal organ. We need to find some indirect approach.

2. The existence of autonomic reflexes: autonomic reflexes are not something we need to think about very much with somatic structures. But visceral pain invokes strong reflexes, usually in the form of smooth-muscle spasm. Can acupuncture have any effect on these reflexes?

Visceral afferents: anatomy and physiology

The afferent nerves from the *viscera* run in autonomic nerves, but in other ways they are similar to somatic nerves, arriving at the substantia gelatinosa of the dorsal horn. Broadly speaking, afferent fibres from, for example, the wall of the gastrointestinal (GI) tract accompany sympathetic nerves and terminate at segments T5 to L1. Some afferent fibres from walls of the lower bowel, bladder other pelvic structures accompany the pelvic plexus (parasympathetic nerves), and terminate at sacral segments (S2–4).

After arriving at the dorsal horn, these afferents project in two directions: firstly, upwards to the autonomic centre in the midbrain and, secondly, within the spinal cord, onto the cell body of the autonomic *efferents* to the organ, which is the basis of the autonomic reflex. These cell bodies are situated in the lateral horn of the spinal cord, shown in Figure 4.3. In the case of the vagal nerve, the equivalent cell bodies are in the vagal nucleus of the medulla. The different spinal segmental levels of the various organs are shown in Table 4.2, and again for reference in the tables in Chapter 16.

The activity of the autonomic cell bodies in the lateral horn is under the control of both the autonomic centre in the hypothalamus and the segmental reflexes from the visceral afferents. There is evidence that acupuncture can influence both systems of control, but here we are interested in the mechanisms in the spinal segment.

Finally, there is one other group of visceral afferent fibres, from the mucosal lining of gut and bladder. These accompany the vagus nerve to the nucleus of the solitary tract in the medulla. This nucleus processes information from several cranial nerves, including taste; but not nociception. It projects to the hypothalamus and to brainstem centres, including the visceromotor and respiratory centres. This system is likely to be involved with generalized physiological and psychological relationships between the senses and the gut.

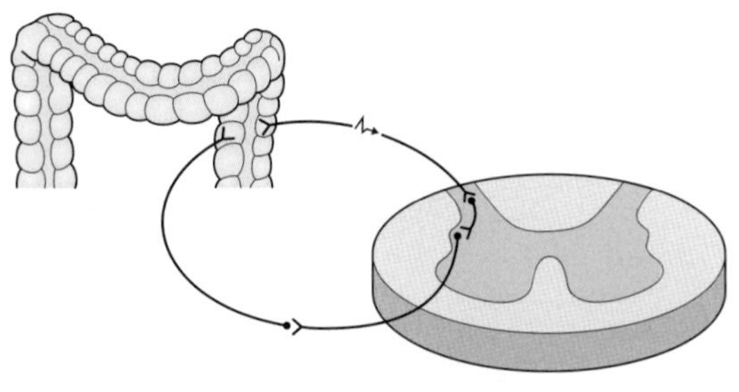

Figure 4.3 Cross section of spinal cord between T1 and L2 showing a visceral afferent nerve synapse in the dorsal horn and project on to the cell body of the autonomic efferent nerve in the lateral grey horn. Note the large amount of white matter (representing nerve fibres travelling longitudinally), indicating that this section is taken high in the thorax.

TABLE 4.2

Levels of autonomic innervation of the viscera

Viscera	Sympathetic	Parasympathetic
Heart	T1 to T5	vagus
Lung and bronchi	T2 to T4	
Oesophagus (caudal part)	T5 to T6	
Stomach	T6 to T10	
Small intestine	T9 to T10	
Large intestine: to splenic flexure	T11 to L1	
Large intestine: splenic flexure to rectum	L1 to L2	S2 to S4
Liver and gall bladder	T7 to T9	vagus
Testis and ovary	T10 to T12	nil
Urinary bladder	T11 to L2	S2 to S4
Uterus	T12 to L1	S2 to S4

Convergence

Each dorsal horn receives afferents from the viscera (such as the bowel) and from somatic structures (the skin and muscles of the abdominal wall). These two afferent pathways *converge* into a single pathway at the dorsal horn, and the brain receives one type of signal, whether somatic or visceral in origin. Therefore, pain from an abdominal organ is perceived as arising in the abdominal wall muscles that have the same segmental innervation. Acupuncturists can exploit convergence to influence the organ by needling the muscle at the same segmental level (Fig. 4.4).

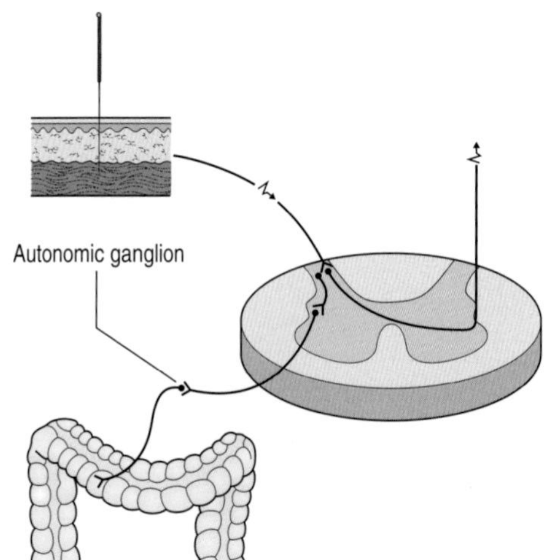

Figure 4.4 Schematic view of convergence: part of the abdominal wall and viscera are supplied by the same segmental level.

The relationship between the muscles and the viscera is reported to operate in both directions, called respectively somatovisceral and viscerosomatic reflexes.

In order to understand how to use these reflex connections in clinical practice, we need to diverge briefly into the embryological development of the human.

Afferent nerves from muscle and organ converge in the dorsal horn.

Segmental development of the foetus

In the early stages of growth of the human foetus its segmental arrangement is very obvious. But as the foetus develops many of the organs and other structures migrate. They drag their nerve supply with them and so they always maintain their original segmental innervation. Different tissues from each segment, such as skin, muscle and viscera, often migrate in different directions. Therefore, in the adult, tissues that are anatomically far apart may be innervated by the same spinal segment. The concept of the '*-tome*' has been introduced to indicate structures that originated at a single segmental level, as shown in Table 4.3.

Autonomic effects of acupuncture

Acupuncture has two kinds of effects on the autonomic nervous system – short term and long term – which are usually in the opposite direction. The moment needles are inserted, they generally evoke a strong sympathetic response in the segment. This can be useful clinically: for example, in acute attacks of hayfever, acupuncture to nearby points can dramatically open the nasal airway by vasoconstricting the nasal mucosa, reducing oedema and inhibiting mucous secretions. The response seems to be related to the strength of stimulation and can continue for some time after treatment.

The long-term sympathetic effects of acupuncture are somewhat different. Since acupuncture depresses the dorsal horn, the result is not only to reduce the perception of pain, but also to produce autonomic blockade by interrupting the autonomic reflexes and reducing smooth-muscle spasm, for example.

TABLE 4.3

Terminology of '-tomes', and their relevance to medical acupuncturists

Tissue	-tome	Relevance
Organ	Viscerotome	Essential to know the segmental origin of the organ; then treatment can be directed at that segment
Skin	Dermatome	Dermatome charts are already well known
Muscles	Myotome	Commonly used, in deep needling of muscles
Periosteum	Sclerotome	Needle accessible areas of bone

Just as the effect on pain accumulates over several sessions, so does the effect on the autonomic reflexes.

Acupuncture may also influence autonomic activity through its effect on higher centres, such as the hypothalamus, which we describe in Chapter 6.

Clinical application to visceral conditions

We now have a rational approach to using acupuncture to treat a visceral problem. Firstly, remember that acupuncture may treat the symptoms, i.e. the pain and autonomic reflexes, but will not change the underlying pathology. Therefore, it is important to know the diagnosis for the correct overall management of the patient.

In choosing a suitable point at which to treat a target organ, first identify at what segmental level the organ is represented (viscerotome) using Table 4.2. Then find a muscle innervated by the same segment (myotome) that you can reach with your needle. There are three groups of muscles you can use:

1. Muscles of the abdominal wall: the choice here is straightforward. Treat where the pain is felt, because this must be the appropriate segment. This also applies in the thorax: treat the muscles (except intercostals) where the pain is felt.
2. Muscles in the paraspinal region: the choice here needs a little more thought. Treat paraspinal muscles at *approximately* the same level as the relevant spinous process. In practice, the longitudinal paraspinal muscles migrate some distance caudally during foetal development, though the short multifidi close to the vertebral column do not. So the latter can be relied on to be situated at their level of origin. The relevant point descriptions in Chapter 16 provide information on innervation of the muscles underlying the points you are likely to use.
3. Muscles in the lower limbs: the choice here needs a little more information. The myotomes of the peripheral acupuncture points cannot be guessed or calculated – we need to know the nerve supply of the underlying muscle. Table 4.4 gives the innervation of some muscles in the leg where common acupuncture points are situated. Do not worry if you do not already know these muscles – they will be like old friends by the time you have been practising acupuncture for a year or two. Again, the innervation of these muscles is presented in the relevant point descriptions in Chapter 16.

TABLE 4.4

Commonly used acupuncture points in the leg, and their innervation

Muscle	Acupuncture point	Myotome
Tibialis anterior	ST36	L4/L5 (S1)
First dorsal interosseus (between hallux and 2nd toe)	LR3	S2/S3
Flexor digitorum longus	SP6	S1/S2

For example, to treat the uterus (S2/S4), we might choose to needle the flexor digitorum longus, the point known as SP6. The standard treatment dose will be the same as that shown in Table 4.1.

In treating the abdominal organs, there are theoretical reasons for preferring to use the points on the abdomen: in laboratory experiments, the response to stimulation of the abdomen is stronger than the response to stimulation elsewhere.

It does not seem possible, in our present state of knowledge, to use specific manipulations of the needle specifically to increase or decrease the autonomic output: acupuncture should probably best be regarded as pushing the reflex response in the direction of normal.

Abdominal organs can be influenced by treating points in the painful area of the abdomen.

It should be noted that we mostly access the sympathetic nerves. The vagus nerve is not accessible to acupuncturists (except, arguably, in the ear, see Chapter 14), and the only accessible parasympathetics are at S2 to S4 levels: these are mainly used for moderating the contraction of detrusor muscle that empties the bladder.

Superficial needling option

While we suggest that intramuscular needling is the standard approach for achieving autonomic effects, other medical acupuncturists find superficial needling perfectly adequate for treating abdominal symptoms. They simply needle the site of the pain.

Summary

Acupuncture stimulates Aδ fibres, whose collateral terminals inhibit the nociceptive pathway in the dorsal horn of the spinal cord. This involves the release of enkephalin. This effect is known as segmental analgesia, and is widely applied in acupuncture treatment of painful areas. Though this treatment is mainly targeting pain relief, its effects seem to bring much wider benefits.

This segmental effect may also be used to influence the symptoms of visceral conditions, both pain and disturbed autonomic reflexes. The afferent pathways of somatic and visceral afferents converge at the dorsal horn, so acupuncture's depressant effect on the dorsal horn applies to both somatic and visceral afferents. Deep intramuscular needling for visceral effects can be given at three sites: muscles of the trunk wall where the pain is felt; paravertebral muscles and muscles in the lower limb that are innervated from the relevant segment. The concept of segmental representation using dermatomes, myotomes, viscerotomes and sclerotomes is useful in planning segmental acupuncture treatment.

Further reading

Bekkering R, van Bussel R 1998 Segmental acupuncture. In Filshie J,White A (eds) Medical acupuncture: a Western scientific approach. Churchill Livingstone, Edinburgh

This chapter gives considerably more detail than our brief introduction, with many useful diagrams, and also provides many supporting references for the concepts and claims made for segmental acupuncture.

CHAPTER

5

Neurological mechanisms III: extrasegmental analgesia

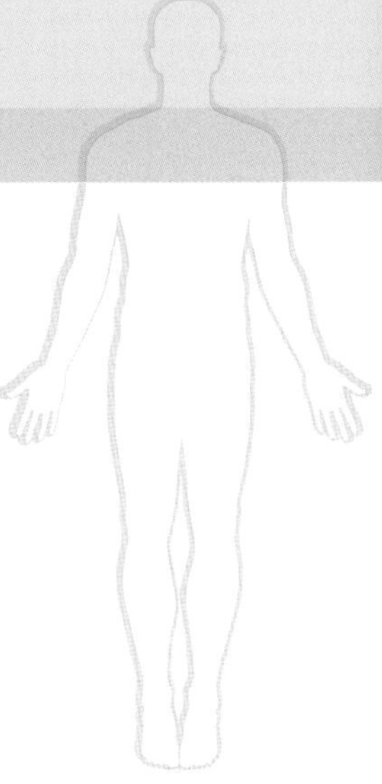

Contents

After reading this chapter you should be able to:

- describe the main sites of β-endorphin and enkephalin release by acupuncture
- summarize the essential features of descending inhibitory pain control.

Introduction

In the previous chapter we discussed the effects of acupuncture on the dorsal horn, which result in segmental analgesia. This effect is used in practice by putting needles somewhere near the painful joint or region, and perhaps in the same limb beyond the painful site – in the same spinal segment as (or one adjacent to) the point at which the noxious input reaches the dorsal horn. However, one well-known feature of acupuncture is the practice of inserting needles some distance away from the painful site – needling the hand to treat the leg, or needling the leg to treat a headache, for example. These needles will probably be stimulated by twirling, possibly several times, and may be left for as long as 20 or 30 minutes. The aim of this manoeuvre is to reinforce the segmental analgesia by activating a more generalized system of analgesia – called extrasegmental analgesia, the subject of this chapter.

This chapter first briefly introduces the biology of opioid peptide release by acupuncture, before going on to describe the mechanisms of extrasegmental analgesia. With this background, the section on clinical application covers the suggested treatment regimens, and then goes on to discuss the mechanisms that explain why different individuals respond differently, why the effect of acupuncture is cumulative, and why you should try to reduce anxiety in patients when you are treating them with acupuncture. Finally, we shall mention the use of acupuncture for surgical analgesia, before closing with a few more general comments on other aspects of pain.

The first report of a proper objective assessment of the analgesia produced by acupuncture was published in 1974, in a study in 60 Chinese medical students. They were given acupuncture at points in the hand (LI4) and knee (ST36) for 50 minutes, after which their threshold to painful electrical stimulation was found to be increased throughout the body – in the head, thorax, back, abdomen and leg (Research Group of Acupuncture Anaesthesia 1974). Another seminal study showed that the analgesia involved a 'humoral factor' (Research Group of Acupuncture Anaesthesia 1974). In this well-known experiment, cerebrospinal fluid (CSF) was drawn from a rabbit that was being given acupuncture and had demonstrated raised pain thresholds. The CSF was perfused into the cerebrospinal space of a second animal, which then developed a similar level of analgesia to the first. Clearly the CSF contained substances that were released by acupuncture, which we now recognize as neuromodulators.

Newer experimental methods have been developed to investigate the neurotransmitters and neuromodulators, and researchers throughout the world have been responsible for exploring the nature of the neurochemical response to acupuncture, but particularly Han in China (Han & Terenius 1982) and Pomeranz in Canada (Pomeranz 2001, Pomeranz & Chiu 1976). More recently, our knowledge of these mechanisms has been extended enormously by the use of magnetic resonance imaging (MRI) techniques, particularly functional MRI (Hui et al 2005, Wu et al 2002), and with positron emission tomography (PET) scanning (Pariente et al 2005).

The advances in our understanding through modern imaging techniques allow us to present a reasonably coherent description of the mechanisms that underlie the central effects of acupuncture, and how these can form a basis for a rational approach to practice. There are of course many gaps in our understanding: for example, many mechanisms of chronic pain are still poorly understood, and our imaging studies are still providing somewhat inconsistent conclusions about the functions of the deeper structures in the brain. Acupuncture seems to have other consistent biological effects and it seems likely that it has other mechanisms awaiting discovery. What we present is, therefore, at best an oversimplification, but enough hopefully to get acupuncture practitioners started on their voyage of discovery.

Neuromodulators: opioid peptides

Acupuncture first gained credibility in the scientific community when it was shown to release naturally occurring opioid peptides. Four opioid peptides have now been identified, but their complete roles in pain perception are still not fully understood (Table 5.1). Each peptide is predominant in a different area

TABLE 5.1

Comparison of properties of the main opioid peptides

Peptide	Main site	Receptor	Blockage by naloxone	Relevant EA frequency (Hz)
β-endorphin	Midbrain, PAG (pituitary)	μ & δ	Low dose	Low (2–4)
Enkephalin	Dorsal horn of spinal cord	μ & δ	Low dose	Low (2–4)
Dynorphin	Brainstem and spine	κ	High dose	High (50–100)
Orphanin	Widespread	μ	Unknown	Low (2–4)

EA = electroacupuncture; Hz = frequency in cycles per second; PAG = peri-aqueductal grey.

of the CNS: *β-endorphin* is found in the brain and *enkephalin* in the spinal cord, and acupuncture causes both to be released. Dynorphin, in the spinal cord and brainstem, has variable effects depending on the circumstances. *Orphanin* (also known as endomorphin or nociceptin) is widely distributed throughout forebrain, midbrain and spinal cord and has a multitude of functions in nociception, other sensory functions and autonomic control (Han 2004).

These opioid peptides are often referred to as neuro*modulators* rather than neuro*transmitters*, because, rather than producing a single response on one occasion only, they have a sustained effect and modify the activity of the target cell over a period of time.

Three types of opioid receptor have been identified, called μ, δ and κ. These are not matched exactly to the different peptides, and some of the peptides stimulate more than one receptor, as shown in Table 5.1.

β-endorphin plays an important role in acupuncture analgesia. In a piece of research that has become a landmark, acupuncture increased the concentrations of β-endorphin in the CSF of patients with pain, whereas control patients who did not receive acupuncture showed no changes (Clement-Jones et al 1980). Subsequent studies have shown that the analgesic effect of acupuncture has a slow onset, reaches a peak after about 20 minutes, and then decays slowly after removing the needles (Fig. 5.1). This time pattern is entirely consistent with the action of neuromodulator release.

The evidence that opioid peptides are involved in acupuncture has been reinforced by the discovery that some of the effects of acupuncture can be reversed by naloxone, both in the laboratory (Han & Terenius 1982, Pomeranz & Chiu 1976) and in clinical trials in patients with pain (Mayer et al 1977). The discovery of specific antagonists to the different receptors has been crucially important in working out the roles of the different opioid peptides.

Acupuncture releases enkephalin in the spinal cord and β-endorphin in the brain.

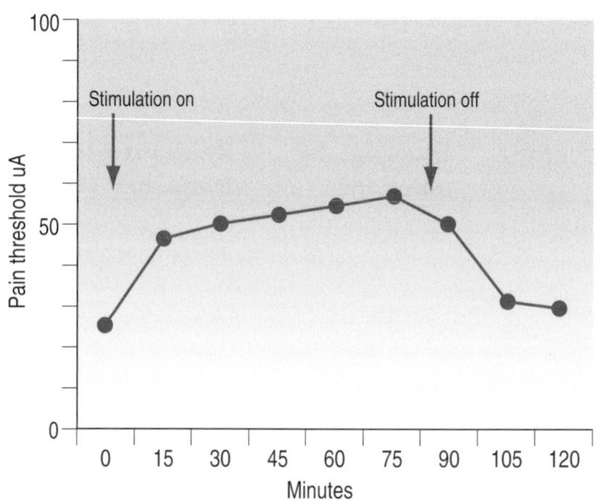

Figure 5.1 Graph indicating changes of dental pain threshold during electrical stimulation to needles in hands and cheeks, showing the delay in rise and fall of analgesia after onset and cessation of acupuncture. (Data from Andersson and Holmgren 1975 American Journal of Chinese Medicine 3(4): 311–334, with permission.)

It is important to note that the discussion above refers to release of the opioid peptides within the CSF. However, β-endorphin is also released from the pituitary directly into the blood stream. This happens in response to several stimuli, not just acupuncture, and the precise role of this circulating β-endorphin in analgesia is not fully understood.

Electroacupuncture and opioid peptides

Electroacupuncture (EA) involves running a small electrical current through needles of sufficient intensity (at least, in laboratory experiments) to make the muscles twitch. Most laboratory research into acupuncture uses EA since it is a reproducible stimulus.

Broadly speaking, different frequencies of EA release different opioid peptides. We owe much of our knowledge on this subject to Ji-Sheng Han, who noticed that acupuncturists vary the way they stimulate needles with spinning or thrusting manoeuvres, sometimes fast and sometimes slow. Han chose the frequencies of 2 Hz and 100 Hz to represent the extremes. He showed that 2 Hz stimulation induces analgesia by release of β-endorphin, enkephalin and orphanin, and their effect on μ receptors; and that high frequency stimulation (typically 80–100 Hz) releases dynorphin, which stimulates κ receptors (see Table 5.1). EA of 15 Hz induces a limited release of both enkephalin and β-endorphin. In a comprehensive review of this laboratory work, Han suggests that the greatest short-term analgesic effect is achieved by combining 2 Hz and 100 Hz (Han 2004). Clinical research in patients with pain has suggested that the effect of 2 Hz is longer lasting than that of 100 Hz (Thomas et al 1995).

Different opioid peptides are released by different stimulation frequencies.

Non-opioid mechanisms in acupuncture analgesia

It has been clear ever since the earliest days of neurophysiological research into acupuncture that the response to needling is complex, and that other transmitters are involved as well as opioids.

Serotonin is one transmitter that is important in the pain control matrix. Serotonin is involved in the brainstem in the activation of the descending pain inhibitory systems, and leads to the release of more serotonin (as well as noradrenaline) in the dorsal horn, as discussed below (Han & Terenius 1982).

Oxytocin may have an important role in many of the effects of acupuncture, including analgesic, anxiolytic and sedative effects (Uvnas-Moberg et al 1993). Oxytocin release is also generated by stroking, gentle massage and physical touch, particularly to the ventral surface of the body.

Analgesia can be produced by shock in some animals. The shock may include painful electrical stimulation in experiments that are supposed to be investigating (non-painful) acupuncture. The mechanism for this effect may be release of ACTH and β-endorphin from the pituitary into the circulation. This can lead to some confusion in interpreting the findings of laboratory studies of electroacupuncture.

Descending inhibitory pain control

In contrast to segmental analgesia described in Chapter 4, acupuncture also induces a generalized analgesia throughout the body. It does this by activating an area in midbrain from which bundles of fibres descend to every level of the spinal cord and inhibit the dorsal horn. The various pathways of descending inhibitory control can be seen in a composite drawing of the neurophysiology of acupuncture (Fig. 5.2).

The crucial structure for this *descending pain inhibition* is the periaqueductal grey (PAG), a small group of cells in the midbrain, and the nearest thing the body has to a 'pain control centre'. The PAG is the site at which the smallest dose of administered opioid drugs (e.g. morphine or heroin) can produce the most profound analgesic effect.

The PAG is activated by β-endorphin, which is released from nerve fibres descending from the hypothalamus, or more precisely the *arcuate nucleus* of the hypothalamus. The arcuate nucleus is also where some of the afferent pathways of the Aδ fibres, stimulated by acupuncture, terminate. (Note that we use the term 'Aδ' to include both the true Aδ fibres in skin and the type II/III fibres in muscle, which acupuncture needles stimulate.) The PAG also receives input from the limbic system, which explains how psychological states can alter the perception of pain.

There are two known descending pathways from the PAG, and probably more that are yet to be discovered:

- One system descending from the PAG releases serotonin at the intermediate cells of the dorsal horn – the same cells that are already activated by the segmental effect of acupuncture. The descending pain control system releases serotonin, stimulating the intermediate cell to release met-enkephalin, which

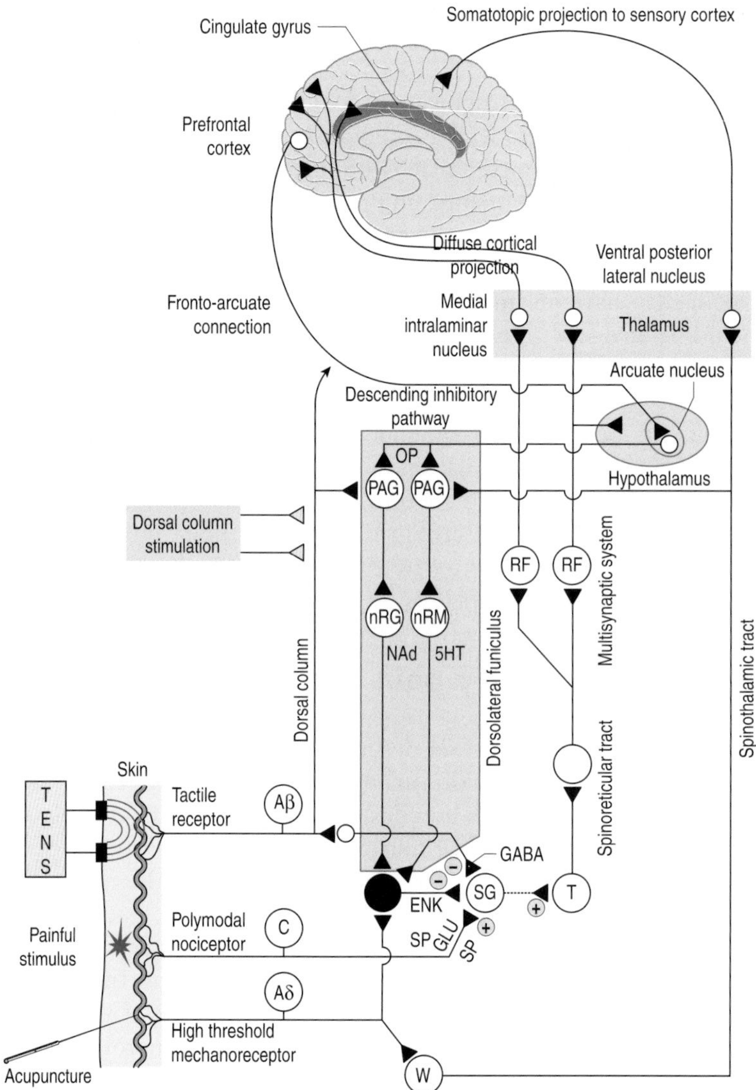

Figure 5.2 Diagram to show neuronal circuits involved in acupuncture and TENS analgesia. The afferent pathways involved in transmitting nociceptive information from a painful scar to the higher centres via the dorsal horn, the ascending tracts and the thalamus are shown. The connections to the descending inhibitory pathways which descend in the dorsolateral funiculus are also shown. The connections to the hypothalamus are indicated. Abbreviations: Aδ, C and Aβ represent the posterior root ganglion cells of small myelinated (A delta) fibres, C fibres and large myelinated fibres, respectively; CGRP = calcitonin gene related peptide; ENK = enkephalinergic neuron; GABA = γ-amino-butyric acid; GLU = glutamate; 5HT = 5-hydroxytryptamine, serotonin; Nad = noradrenaline = norepinephrine; nRG = nucleus raphe gigantocellularis; nRM = nucleus raphe magnus; OP = opioid peptides; PAG = periaqueductal grey; RF = reticular formation; SG = cell in the substantia gelatinosa; SP = substance P; T = transmission cell; VIP = vasoactive intestinal polypeptide; W = Waldeyer cell; + = stimulant effect; − = inhibitory effect. (From Filshie and Thompson 2004 The Oxford Book of Palliative Medicine. 3rd edn. Chapter 8.2.9. Reproduced with permission of Oxford University Press.)

in turn inhibits the substantial gelatinosa cells (see Fig. 5.2). This effect will be in addition to any segmental inhibition that is already active.

- Another descending pathway causes the release of noradrenaline diffusely throughout the dorsal horn. Noradrenaline has a direct inhibitory effect on the post-synaptic membrane of the transmission cells, further reinforcing the effect of acupuncture on controlling nociception (Figs 5.3 & 5.4).

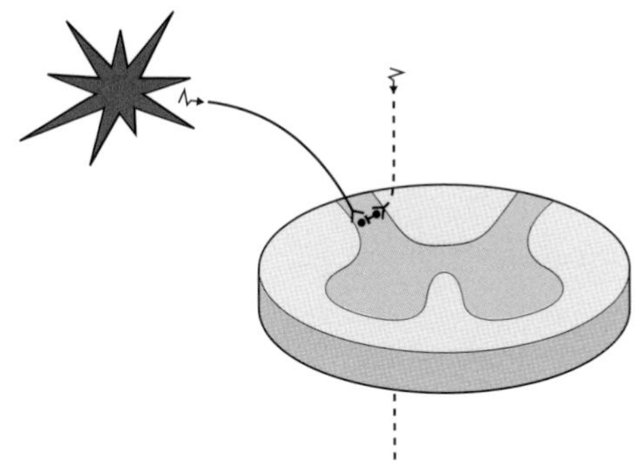

Figure 5.3 Descending pain inhibition by release of serotonin modulating intermediate cells.

Descending inhibitory pain control inhibits the nociceptive pathway in every dorsal horn.

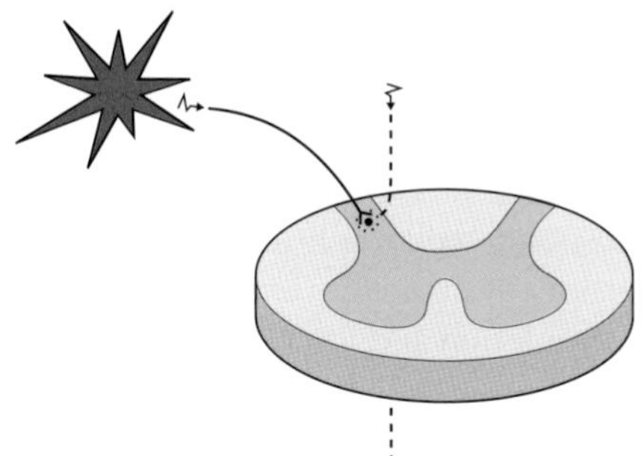

Figure 5.4 Descending pain inhibition by release of noradrenaline around substantia gelatinosa cells.

These particular actions of acupuncture might be influenced by pharmacological intervention. For example, tricyclic antidepressant drugs increase the release of both serotonin and noradrenaline in the central nervous system; there is some (admittedly not strong) evidence that tricyclic antidepressants may be synergistic with acupuncture and increase its analgesic effect. Interestingly, this effect is not seen with the selective serotonin reuptake inhibitory drugs.

Clinical application

Extrasegmental acupuncture can be used to reinforce segmental analgesia. Point selection is not likely to be critical because this is a generalized affect throughout the body. Extrasegmental analgesia can probably be generated

TABLE 5.2

Standard dose of acupuncture for extrasegmental analgesia (in addition to needling for segmental analgesia)

Variable	Typical of standard treatment
Points	In limbs, usually bilateral
Number of needles	Typically two or four
Depth of insertion	Intramuscular
Needle stimulation	Manual, or electrical using low and high frequencies
Response elicited	*de qi*, muscle contraction if electroacupuncture
Needle retention time	20 minutes

most effectively at the well-known major acupuncture points such as LI4 or LI11 in the arms, and ST36 or LR3 in the legs.

The standard dose of acupuncture needed for extrasegmental analgesia is shown in Table 5.2 – this can be applied in addition to any needles used for segmental analgesia, though still having respect for each individual person's sensitivity to acupuncture. Electrical stimulation is probably more effective than manual for activating this particular effect of acupuncture.

For a sustained effect in treating chronic pain, repeat the stimulus once or twice a week so that the benefit accumulates, for reasons discussed below.

Individual response to acupuncture

Patients vary considerably in their response to acupuncture. Some patients respond well to brief, superficial needling, and may experience ill-effects from any stronger treatment. Others fail to respond to even strong, prolonged stimulation and are classified as 'non-responders'. The majority of the population lies somewhere in between these two extremes and responds in a way that we can recognize as 'normal'.

This variation in response is likely to be due to genetic differences in patients' opioid peptide metabolism, and differences in receptor activity. In laboratory experiments, genetic differences between animals can mean that up to 50% of some batches of animal fail to respond to needling stimulation in the expected way. Another reason for different individual responses is likely to be variation in the activity of the enzyme enkephalinase in the spinal cord.

Cumulative response to acupuncture: gene expression

In treating many painful conditions with acupuncture, relief of pain usually accumulates gradually over a series of treatments. This may be explained by changes in opioid peptide metabolism. Any stimulus that leads to the release of opioid peptides also enhances gene expression so that more opioid peptide is manufactured and stored at the terminal; next time the stimulus is applied it releases more peptide. This increased gene expression needs to be reinforced within a short period of time or it will decay back to normal. The optimal interval may be about 3 days, although in clinical practice it is often difficult to arrange treatments this frequently.

The effect of acupuncture accumulates when it is repeated.

Natural opioid antagonist cholecystokinin: anxiety

Cholecystokinin (CCK) is a naturally occurring antagonist of opioid peptides. It was named after being first found to cause contraction of the gall bladder. Raised levels of CCK in the CNS are associated with an increased perception of pain; in addition, anxious patients have raised levels of CCK and, therefore, are likely to experience more pain.

Therefore, to achieve the maximal benefit from opioid release, it is important to prepare patients for acupuncture in ways that reduce anxiety, such as avoiding rush, providing adequate explanation, leaving opportunities for questions and discussion, as well as using touch, if appropriate. Apart from being good practice anyway, a relaxed patient will have lower levels of CCK and better results with acupuncture theoretically.

In addition, it is worth remembering that CCK is released by acupuncture stimulation in the laboratory when it is prolonged for more than about 45 minutes. Acupuncture analgesia for postoperative pain control or for labour pain may need to be continued for more than 2 hours. Theoretically this continued stimulation could become counterproductive, though several studies have suggested that this is not a significant problem clinically.

Acupuncture analgesia for surgery

The combined effects of segmental and extrasegmental acupuncture stimulation have been used as the basis for acupuncture analgesia (or, more strictly speaking, *hyp*algesia – reduced pain) for surgery. The increase in pain threshold that can be achieved by acupuncture in any particular patient varies greatly with many factors, including, for example, the particular circumstances and the susceptibility of the individual. While dramatic early reports from China showed major surgery apparently being conducted using acupuncture as the main form of analgesia, subsequent experience suggests that few individuals achieve sufficient increase in pain threshold to permit surgery. In practice, acupuncture analgesia when used alone for surgery is unreliable and not considered worthwhile as a sole intervention.

Aspects of pain

Classification of pain

It is important for acupuncturists to try to recognize what type of pain their patient has, from history and examination, because not all types respond reliably to treatment. In practice, of course, it is often difficult to be sure, and many patients with chronic pain have features of more than one type of pain.

Nociceptive pain is the result of stimulation of the peripheral nerves – e.g. from tissue damage, degeneration, inflammation or ischaemia. Nociceptive pain is common, and examples include the pain of healing from injury, the pain of arthritic joints and myofascial pain. This type of pain is generally likely to respond to acupuncture, and to have a cumulative response to repeated treatment.

Neuropathic pain is caused by abnormal function of the nervous system, either caused by trauma or as part of a neurological condition. The abnormality may be peripheral or central or both: examples include post-herpetic neuralgia, phantom limb pain, post-stroke pain and complex regional pain syndrome. Patients often describe neuropathic pain with characteristic adjectives ('shooting' or 'burning'), and they may show allodynia (pain caused by a normally pain-free stimulus like brushing the skin) and hyperalgesia (severe pain from minor noxious stimulus). Since the nervous system is itself damaged, it is hardly surprising that acupuncture is often less helpful for patients with neuropathic pain. In addition, there is a slight risk that acupuncture will exacerbate neuropathic pain if it is not given correctly.

Chronic pain of any origin is often complicated by *psychological* aspects, such as depression and fear avoidance, though pain of purely psychological origin is extremely rare. The role of acupuncture in blocking the psychological aspects of pain is unpredictable, but it may have other effects that are useful to the patient such as improved sleep. The response to any treatment depends in part on the patient's beliefs and expectations and the strength of the therapeutic relationship, as well as any specific effects on the pain pathways. Acupuncture may contribute usefully to recovery within a pain management strategy that also includes information, modification of treatment objectives, and exercise.

In a primary-care setting of civilian and military populations (Cummings 1996), the response rates to acupuncture for different types of pain were as follows:

- 90% in patients with myofascial pain
- 70% in patients with other forms of nociceptive pain
- 40% in other types of pain.

Acupuncture is most predictably effective for treating nociceptive pain.

Sensitization: peripheral and central

In certain circumstances, a patient's response to a noxious stimulus can be amplified out of proportion to the degree of injury or pathology that seems to be present. For example, a joint that is inflamed may be extremely tender to the lightest touch, or a limb that has recovered from injury may remain

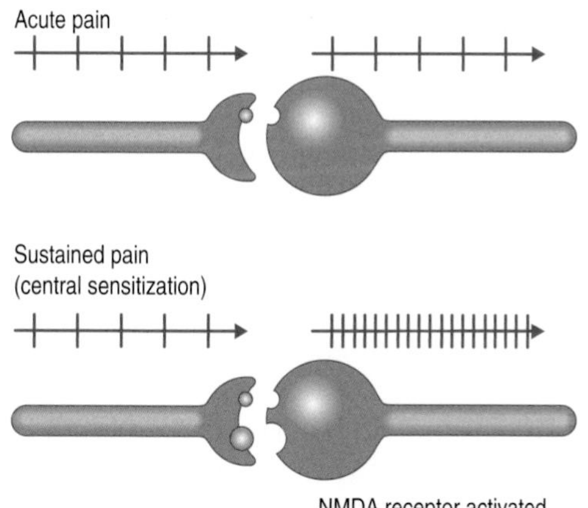

Figure 5.5 Schematic drawing of central sensitization, showing the standard response of the pathway to acute pain, and the heightened response in chronic pain when the second receptor is activated.

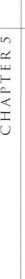

unduly sensitive. In these cases, sensitization has occurred, which can be either peripheral or central or both:

- Peripheral sensitization: the sensory nerve endings are sensitized by inflammatory mediators released locally and they respond strongly to even a minor stimulus.
- Central sensitization: if a nociceptive stimulus is repeated, the response of some spinal cord transmission cells becomes more vigorous, a process called 'wind up' (Woolf 1996), and shown schematically in Figure 5.5. Sensitization results from the recruitment of a second glutamate receptor, previously dormant, the 'NMDA' receptor. In chronic pain this receptor is activated semi-permanently, which is then referred to as central sensitization. Activation of the NMDA receptor results in a much greater response to stimulation than the basic 'AMPA' receptor, which is the one that first responds to the release of glutamate from a primary nociceptive afferent nerve. Similar mechanisms may operate in other sites throughout the CNS pathway and lead to further amplification of the pain.

Tenderness throughout the body may indicate central sensitization.

Strong stimulation: diffuse noxious inhibitory control

One further concept should be mentioned for the sake of completeness. Strong stimulation anywhere in the body may produce 'diffuse noxious inhibitory control' or DNIC, a widespread pain inhibition involving the descending mechanisms mentioned above (Le Bars et al 1979). In laboratory experiments, the effect has a rapid onset but is short-lived, only lasting about twice the duration of the stimulation. Stimulation this strong is rarely used in clinical practice in the West.

Summary

Neuromodulators of the opioid peptide group have been shown to be involved in acupuncture analgesia. Electrical stimulation at different frequencies stimulates the release of different peptides. Acupuncture can induce widespread relief of pain by stimulating the endogenous system known as descending inhibitory pain control. Through local release of β-endorphin in the periaqueductal grey, at least two descending tracts are activated that inhibit the transmission of nociceptive pathways in the dorsal horn, at every segmental level. The transmitters released locally in the dorsal horn are serotonin and noradrenaline. The biology of the opioid peptides goes some way to explaining why individual patients respond to acupuncture differently, why the effects of acupuncture accumulate, and why patients should be relaxed when they are given acupuncture. Acupuncture analgesia is not reliable enough on its own for surgery.

Pain is generally classified into nociceptive or neurogenic, and both have psychological components. Acupuncture is most effective against nociceptive pain. The nervous system can be sensitized to nociception, either peripherally where the responsiveness of nerves is increased by the presence of inflammatory mediators, or centrally where additional receptors are recruited that amplify the nociceptive signal.

Further reading

Melzack R, Wall P D 1982 The challenge of pain. Penguin Science, Harmondsworth

This highly accessible book written by the originators of the gate control theory of pain gives a masterful insight into modern concepts of how the body handles pain.

The following selection of scientific reviews describe classic milestones in the evolution of the understanding of mechanisms of action of acupuncture, and are generally highly accessible overviews that provide extensive reference lists:

Andersson S, Lundeberg T 1995 Acupuncture – from empiricism to science: functional background to acupuncture effects in pain and disease. Medical Hypotheses 45: 271–281

Bowsher D 1998 Mechanisms of acupuncture. In Filshie J, White A (eds) Medical acupuncture: a Western scientific approach. Churchill Livingstone, Edinburgh, pp 69–82

Carlsson C 2002 Acupuncture mechanisms for clinically relevant long-term effects – reconsideration and a hypothesis. Acupuncture in Medicine 20: 82–99

Han J, Terenius L 1982 Neurochemical basis of acupuncture analgesia. Annual Reviews in Pharmacology and Toxicology 22: 193–220

Han J S 1997 Physiology of acupuncture: review of thirty years of research. Journal of Alternative and Complementary Medicine 3(Suppl 1): S101–S108

Han J S 2004 Acupuncture and endorphins. Neuroscience Letters 361: 258–261

Pomeranz B 2001 Acupuncture analgesia – basic research. In Stux G, Hammerschlag R (eds) Clinical acupuncture – scientific basis. Springer, Berlin

CHAPTER

6

Neurological mechanisms IV: central regulatory effects

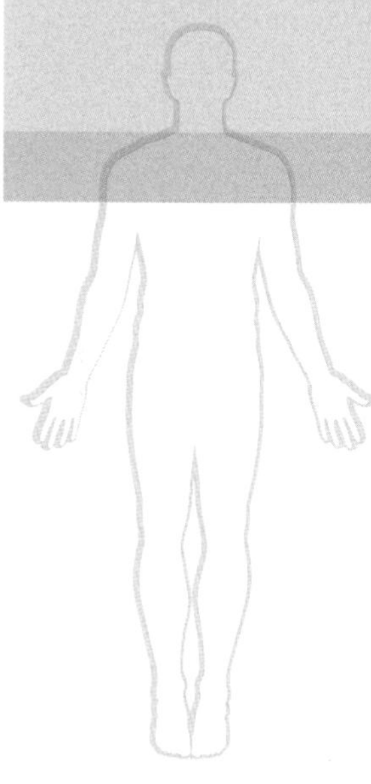

Contents

After reading this chapter, you should be able to:

- give a brief overview of the limbic system
- name at least four central regulatory functions that may be influenced by acupuncture.

Introduction

One of the things that make acupuncture so satisfying is hearing patients report the unexpected benefits of treatment. They not only report the expected relief of pain – sometimes for the first time – but they also frequently state that they felt calm and relaxed, and slept unusually well after treatment. The words that different patients use are remarkably consistent, though of course not all patients do experience these things. Acupuncturists and their patients are in no doubt that acupuncture can have profound and widespread physiological effects.

We shall use the term 'central regulatory' effects for these rather general changes: 'central' because they clearly take place in the central nervous system, and 'regulatory' because they seem to be stabilizing effects, moving the body towards normal function – in terms of arousal or sleep, for example. There is evidence that these effects occur reproducibly, although their mechanisms are not yet entirely clear and this chapter relies rather more than the others on a degree of extrapolation – clinical observations interpreted by plausible suggestions of mechanisms for which there is partial evidence, but not complete proof. As a result, the advice on treatment techniques is less secure than other chapters. But even if the precise mechanisms turn out to be rather different from those we describe here, we believe that these effects are important enough to be included in standard texts of acupuncture in the hope and expectation that new insights into CNS function will provide more solid explanations in the future.

Pain: the affective component

Pain has a *sensory* component – its nature, quality and duration – which is registered at the somatosensory cortex, and an *affective* component – its emotional aspect; how disturbing it is – which is registered in the limbic system.

A patient might describe a pain that is mainly sensory like this: 'It hurts me, but it doesn't disturb me very much, I can handle it'. It is the sensory component that segmental and extrasegmental acupuncture treat through their effects on the dorsal horn.

A patient who has a painful condition with a strong *affective* component finds it profoundly disturbing. A headache, for example, often appears to incapacitate a patient more than the level of pain itself would seem to warrant. Pain is obviously more than a sensation, it is an unpleasant experience and it has many dimensions: basically, the sensation has to be processed so that avoiding action can be organized. At a cognitive level, a new pain experience needs to be compared with previous experiences (memory) so that it can be interpreted (reasoning) and evaluated (judgement): but, in evolutionary terms, survival may also depend on activating appropriate reactions including an emotional response and physical responses, such as autonomic changes.

The limbic system

Many of these aspects of processing and responding to pain are the responsibility of the *limbic system*, an interconnected group of structures lying deep within the brain. The limbic system includes the amygdala, hippocampus, parahippocampus, anterior cingulate cortex (ACC), prefrontal cortex, septum, nucleus accumbens, hypothalamus, insula and caudate. A simplified scheme was shown in Figure 4.2, and some of the responses to acupuncture are shown in Plate 5.

There is now good evidence from imaging studies that acupuncture has a considerable effect on the limbic system (Hui et al 2000, Hui et al 2005, Pariente et al 2005). This is a rather general effect of acupuncture, and almost certainly does not depend on the needle site, but rather on a combination of factors including the stimulus and, to a certain extent, the patient's belief and expectations.

Interestingly, there is now rather good evidence that a convincing form of sham acupuncture (using blunt needles, but suggesting to the patient that this is an active treatment) can produce distinct changes in the limbic system. It seems highly probable that the Aδ fibres usually stimulated by acupuncture are not involved in conveying this effect, and it is much more likely that this effect of sham acupuncture on the limbic system is a result of touch activating the C tactile fibre system (Lund & Lundeberg 2006). These aspects of treatment could be described as the pleasantness of acupuncture. With genuine acupuncture, when needles are inserted and stimulated in an appropriate way, there is an additional effect that seems to involve the insula very specifically.

The limbic system is responsible for the affective component of pain.

Another study has shown that gentle needling at ST36, enough to elicit *de qi* but not sharp pain, caused a reduction in the magnetic resonance imaging (MRI) signal intensity throughout the limbic system (Hui et al 2005). A reduced signal may indicate lower neuronal activity, though that is not absolutely clear. The reduction was most marked in the amygdala, hippocampus, parahippocampus, anterior cingulate cortex (ACC) and prefrontal cortex; and was significant, but more limited, in the septal area, nucleus accumbens, hypothalamus, insula and caudate. The dorsal raphe nucleus showed increased activity and, since this nucleus projects to the periaqueductal grey, the finding is compatible with activation of the descending inhibitory pain system by acupuncture, as discussed in Chapter 5. In contrast, acupuncture that produced a sensation of sharp pain and *de qi* produced a mixture of signal changes, with some activation and some decrease. Though our knowledge of the exact mechanisms is still limited, the evidence is accumulating that acupuncture – at least under certain conditions – can have useful effects on the limbic system.

One interpretation of this evidence from imaging studies is that the affective component of pain will respond to any form of acupuncture that stimulates the limbic system, whereas the sensory component of pain is likely to respond better to the specific analgesic effects of segmental and extrasegmental acupuncture. The limbic system can be stimulated by rather non-specific needling, whereas segmental analgesia depends more on eliciting *de qi* in the appropriate segment. This difference could explain the findings of the large series of clinical trials in Germany in the early 2000s: acupuncture and sham acupuncture have similar effects on migraine, tension headache and back pain, whereas for knee pain segmental acupuncture is significantly superior to sham acupuncture. The explanation that has been proposed is that migraine, tension headache and back pain have a high affective component, which responds to non-specific needle stimulation (Lund & Lundeberg 2006). In contrast, knee pain is mainly sensory, so specific analgesic effects are required.

The affective component of pain is rarely measured in clinical trials, but at least one study has found that patients who have received acupuncture report that the affective component is reduced more than the sensory component (Thomas et al 1991). Patients may still have their chronic pain, but it bothers them less.

Psychological changes

Acupuncture treatment may be associated with several profound mental effects:

- Commonly, a rather general emotional calming, with a sense of euphoria, peace and relaxation, which some patients describe as 'wholeness' or 'balance'
- A good night's sleep, particularly after the first one or two treatments with acupuncture
- Occasionally, quite strong emotional reactions to treatment, such as weeping or giggling and, occasionally, anger
- Uncommonly other events such as fainting, and, extremely rarely, reactions such as seizure or temporary comatose states.

This general improvement in wellbeing can be particularly valuable for patients with chronic pain. Not only is the pain less bothersome, but they feel better equipped to cope with it. These changes seem not to be dependent on any specific point locations, though they may be more marked after needling major points. This difference has been noticed in acupuncture training courses, where novices treat each other intensively for practice. Drowsiness seems more common after needling the major points than after needling trigger points in muscle.

Autonomic effects

Acupuncture can cause generalized sympathetic responses in different directions. In the short term, tone is increased locally in the segment during treatment, and in the long term there is evidence of a widespread, sustained decrease in sympathetic tone. In general, low-frequency electrical stimulation reduces tone and high frequency increases it, at least in laboratory studies. There is good evidence from laboratory studies that acupuncture can alter autonomic activity at the level of the hypothalamus (as well as the dorsal horn, which we discussed earlier), and this matches the changes observed clinically.

The effect of acupuncture on the organism depends on the current status of the autonomic balance. For example, some studies have shown that acupuncture can, in the short term, reduce a raised blood pressure and increase a low blood pressure. While studies have shown no long-term benefit of acupuncture for hypertension, for reasons that are not clear, the effect can be clinically useful for other conditions when autonomic outflow is functionally disturbed, for example in treatment of functional bladder disorders. The decreased sympathetic tone can be reinforced by repeat treatment (Dyrehag et al 1997). Some evidence also suggests that acupuncture can have some effect on conditions that are sympathetic-dependent, such complex regional pain syndrome and Raynaud's disease.

Hypothalamo–pituitary–adrenal axis

Acupuncture stimulation may influence the anterior pituitary gland via the hypothalamus. There is evidence that it stimulates the release into the circulation of both ACTH and β-endorphin, which are derived from a single precursor, pro-opiomelanocortin. How relevant the increased circulation of ACTH and β-endorphin after acupuncture are in clinical practice is not clear, since β-endorphin does not cross the blood–brain barrier. β-endorphin concentrations in the blood also respond to many non-specific stimuli, such as eating and exercise. It is important to distinguish this β-endorphin circulating in the blood stream from that which is released within the CNS around the periaqueductal grey.

Hypothalamo–pituitary–ovarian axis

The arcuate nucleus of the hypothalamus is the site for the so-called gonadotrophin (GnRH) pulse generator, so it is not unreasonable to predict that acupuncture may have some effect on release of GnRH. The clinical effects of this could include alteration in the regulation of menstrual timing and flow, and reduction of dysmenorrhoea. These effects on gonadotrophin releasing hormone are now established, but the clinical effects, though reported widely as anecdotes, are not firmly supported by clinical trials.

Other endocrine effects

Postmenopausal hot flushes are due to dysfunction of the temperature regulatory centre, though the mechanism is not currently known. Some evidence suggests that release of β-endorphin tends to reduce the frequency of hot flushes, possibly by modifying the activity of CGRP, which is a potent vasodilator (Wyon et al 1995), or by release of 5-HT, which has an effect on thermoregulation. Small clinical trials have suggested that acupuncture may reduce the incidence or severity of postmenopausal flushes, but it is still unclear whether this is more than an effect of expectation.

There are anecdotal reports that some patients find they need to alter their dose of insulin for a few days after having acupuncture, though there is little reliable evidence that acupuncture can have any useful clinical effect on insulin-dependent diabetic patients.

The immune system

The mechanisms of activation and control of the immune system have only relatively recently been understood in any great depth. Acupuncture has been found in some studies to enhance the immune system (Lundeberg 1999). Possible mechanisms include generalized or localized autonomic changes regulating the lymphoreticular system in the bone marrow and spleen, or circulation of β-endorphin, which induces immune changes through receptors on leukocytes. It is still not clear whether these effects of acupuncture are clinically relevant.

Drug dependency

Acupuncture has gained a reputation for helping addicts withdraw from their drugs. Acupuncture can reduce the excess dopamine production in the nucleus accumbens, which is the common pathway for addiction (Yoon et al 2004). There are probably two separate clinical effects: a short-term reduction of the withdrawal symptoms, and an improvement in the person's attitude and motivation making them more likely to participate in the appropriate counselling and support services. Studies that simply test the effect on withdrawal alone have been disappointing, though they have often involved inadequate stimulation. The claims that acupuncture can motivate addicts to engage in conventional treatment programmes have not yet been tested.

Nausea and vomiting

One of the clinical areas where controlled clinical studies of acupuncture were first, convincingly and repeatedly, positive is nausea and vomiting, whether due to pregnancy, surgery or chemotherapy. These early studies have been followed by many others from different centres, generally confirming the effect. The sensation of nausea is a response of the emetic centre and chemoreceptor zones to a variety of stimuli. Acupuncture, usually given at a point in the wrist (PC6), on the upper abdomen (CV12) or one below the knee (ST36), reduces the emetic response, but the precise mechanisms of action are still unknown.

Clinical application

The effects discussed in this chapter are seen after treatment at the major points, mostly in the hands and feet, and particularly ST36 just below the knee. Although traditional Chinese acupuncturists apparently used individualized points according to the patient's history and typology, the evidence suggests that the effects we describe in this chapter are rather generalized responses to acupuncture, and not specific effects of any particular points. The *nature* of the stimulus (the dose of acupuncture) may well be more relevant than *where* it is given. Auricular acupuncture may be useful for inducing central regulatory effects, as discussed in Chapter 14.

It is difficult to predict the response of any individual patient, so practitioners must learn to observe carefully how the patient responds, and to adjust the dose of acupuncture accordingly. Responses can be powerful, and practitioners should be aware of unwanted emotional effects. Patients who appear in any way emotionally unstable should be treated particularly carefully, and a course of treatment should not be prolonged in these patients if their condition does not resolve quickly.

To maximize these central effects, it seems important to ensure that the nervous system is appropriately 'primed' before treatment: this means that the patient should be relaxed, confident, warm and comfortable, if at all possible. After inserting the needles, let the patient relax quietly for 10 to 30 minutes without disturbance.

Many of the laboratory studies exploring these central effects have used electrical stimulation of needles, though in clinical practice manual acupuncture is much more common. It may be sensible to consider electroacupuncture if there is no response to manual stimulation. The 'standard treatment template' for this approach would look something like that shown in Table 6.1.

Summary

This chapter describes the mechanisms of action which underlie some beneficial effects of needling not already covered. Pain may have a strong affective component involving the limbic system, and acupuncture can influence the

TABLE 6.1

Standard acupuncture treatment for central effects

Variable	Typical of standard treatment
Points	Major points in limbs, or possibly auricular points
Number of needles	Two or three bilaterally
Depth of insertion	Deep, usually intramuscular (superficial in auricular points)
Needle stimulation	Gentle manual stimulation, once or twice; or sometimes electrical stimulation
Response elicited	*De qi*, or muscle contraction if using electrical stimulation
Needle retention time	10–30 minutes

(Caution: this type of treatment may also cause drowsiness and patients should not drive afterwards if they are affected.)

limbic system. Its effect on the affective component of pain is likely to be separate from the effect on the sensory component that is obtained by the specific analgesic effects of segmental and extrasegmental acupuncture. Acupuncture may have other regulatory effects on various functions, including mood and motivation, autonomic effects, the hypothalamo–pituitary–adrenal axis, the hypothalamo–pituitary–ovarian axis and the immune system. Central mechanisms also underlie acupuncture's role in treating drug-dependency and nausea and vomiting.

CHAPTER 7

Myofascial trigger points

Contents

After reading this chapter you should be able to:

- describe the essential features of myofascial trigger points
- list four major diagnostic criteria
- describe the pain referral pattern of two myofascial trigger points.

Introduction

The one type of acupuncture treatment that we have not yet discussed involves the practitioner examining a muscle to find its most tender point and needling that point precisely. He or she then stimulates the needle, and may withdraw it straightaway. Sometimes, the patient experiences immediate relief of pain. We believe that acupuncture is most rapidly effective for a particular type of tender point called a *myofascial trigger point* (MTrP). It is not unreasonable to speculate that acupuncture may have been developed originally as a treatment for these MTrPs.

Muscles form the largest organ in the body. They usually recover rapidly from injury, but occasionally they develop a tender and hyperirritable spot, the MTrP. This causes persistent pain, which has certain characteristics that can help distinguish it from other painful conditions. This chapter discusses all aspects of the MTrP, and is the final chapter on the mechanisms of Western medical acupuncture.

The two authors who have made the greatest contribution to the understanding of trigger points are Travell and Simons, physicians from rheumatology and pain-management backgrounds in conventional medicine (Simons et al 1999, Travell & Simons 1983, Travell & Simons 1992). Their rigorous approach to the diagnosis, mechanisms and treatment of MTrPs established them as a clinical condition and separated them from a confusing rag-bag of doubtful or non-committal diagnoses in soft-tissue pain disorders, such as fibrositis, myalgia and muscular rheumatism.

Many conventional healthcare practitioners are unfamiliar with the MTrP and have difficulty accepting it as a condition. Even physicians specializing in orthopaedics or rheumatology often dismiss MTrP pain, either because the condition is not common in the type of patient they see, or because they regard the whole subject of soft-tissue pain as a 'grey area' consisting of borderline diagnoses linked to psychological problems and dismiss it all as 'functional'.

There is now considerable accumulated clinical experience in treating the MTrP, and the evidence in support of the MTrP as a genuine clinical entity is marked by the following milestones:

- Pain arising from muscles is referred. In an extensive series of experiments, Kellgren injected himself and his colleagues with hypertonic saline: injections into most soft tissues produced local pain, but injections into muscle consistently caused pain to be referred at a distance (Kellgren 1938). This has been amply confirmed in many studies since that time.
- MTrPs continuously generate spontaneous electrical activity of very low voltage (Hubbard & Berkoff 1993).
- The diagnosis of MTrPs can be made reliably by blinded examiners – if they are appropriately trained (Gerwin et al 1997).
- A hypothesis for a mechanism has been proposed (Mense & Simons 1999).
- MTrPs show greater density of immunoreactivity to substance P (a nociceptive neurotransmitter) compared with normal muscle (De Stefano et al 2000).
- The precise location of MTrPs can be identified reliably by two examiners independently (Sciotti et al 2001).
- Extracellular fluid surrounding an MTrP and collected by micro-dialysis (Shah et al 2005) contains higher concentrations than normal of several known nociceptor compounds that sensitize high-threshold nerve fibres in muscle. These compounds include protons (H+), bradykinin, calcitonin gene-related peptide, substance P, tumour-necrosis factor-α, interleukin 1-β, serotonin and noradrenaline (norephinephrine).

Many practitioners only discover MTrPs when they learn acupuncture; some describe it as a revelation in their medical practice, especially in primary care, as they are now able to diagnose and treat many patients who were previously classified rather unsatisfactorily as 'functional', and perhaps dismissed as impossible to diagnose or treat.

Although MTrPs were described by Travell and Simons within the context of conventional medicine, they do seem to correlate rather well with aspects of traditional Chinese acupuncture. Common trigger points are often situated at known acupuncture points, and one landmark study found 100% correlation between MTrPs and acupuncture points (Melzack et al 1977). Traditional acupuncturists have been using *ah shi* points for many years: an *ah shi* point is one which, when pressed, causes the patient involuntarily to shout out *ah shi*, which means 'Oh yes!' ('... that is my pain'). In addition, many of the traditional acupuncture meridians are strikingly similar to the patterns of referred pain from trigger points.

MTrPs are an example of how the best of complementary and conventional approaches can be integrated; a significant step forward in patient care.

Definition

Travell and Simons defined an MTrP as a 'hyperirritable locus within a taut band of skeletal muscle, located in the muscle tissue or its associated fascia' (Travell & Simons 1983).

An MTrP is a hyperirritable locus within a taut band of skeletal muscle.

The essential clinical features of an MTrP are:

- a taut band can be palpated inside the belly of the muscle
- part of the taut band is very tender
- pressing that tender spot causes pain that the patient recognizes
- movement of the joint that stretches the muscle is restricted by pain.

Pressure on an MTrP replicates the patient's pain when pressed.

An MTrP may be *active* and cause stiffness and pain, or *latent* and cause stiffness without pain. An active MTrP may be inactivated by treatment, and a latent MTrP may be activated by a number of precipitating factors, described in Mechanisms.

MTrPs tend to occur in rather constant positions within muscles, for example the anterior border of the upper fibres of trapezius (Fig. 7.1). Our diagrams mark the trigger point with cross hatches (with the long strokes in the direction of the fibres) and the pain either in colour, or with cross hatching.

Many points in the body are tender: only MTrPs have the characteristic features.

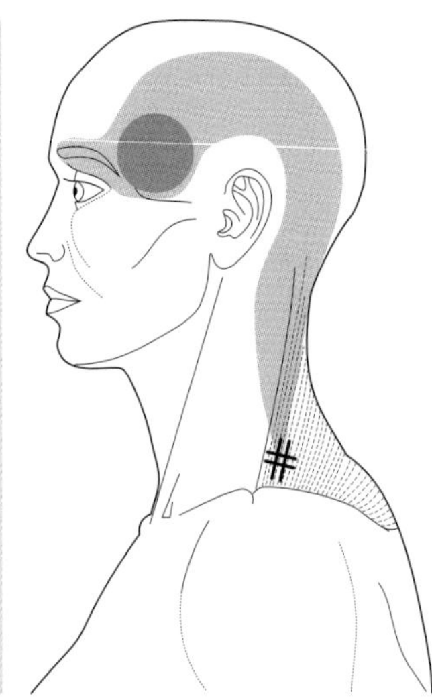

Figure 7.1 Trigger point in upper fibres of trapezius referring pain mainly to the neck and temporal region.

Incidence

MTrPs are common, and most people develop one or more during their lifetime. Physicians who are experienced in identifying trigger points could find at least one MTrP in about half of healthy, symptom-free young service personnel (Sola et al 1955). In one study in primary care, MTrPs were found in 30% of patients consulting for pain (Skootsky et al 1989). However, in reality they are not likely to be the *primary* cause of pain as frequently as this.

Aetiology

MTrPs may be caused by muscle injury or strain, but they may also occur secondary to other painful conditions. A strain that causes an MTrP in one patient may not bother a second patient – or even the same patient at another time, suggesting that there are other factors that make MTrPs more likely to develop. The same factors may prevent them healing.

Myofascial trigger points from acute or chronic muscle strain

Trigger points may arise rapidly in the few days following an acute strain of the muscle, or they may arise insidiously following chronic strain.

Most MTrPs are caused by muscle injury – acute or chronic.

The commonest acute strain occurs when the muscle is overloaded, for example from lifting something too heavy, or at an awkward angle. One muscle that is vulnerable to sudden overuse strain is pectoralis major (Fig. 7.2), commonly in young men with heavy occupations. Quadratus lumborum (Fig. 7.3), which is crucial in providing lateral support for the back, can easily be strained lifting a weight with one hand. In these cases, the onset of pain is usually rapid.

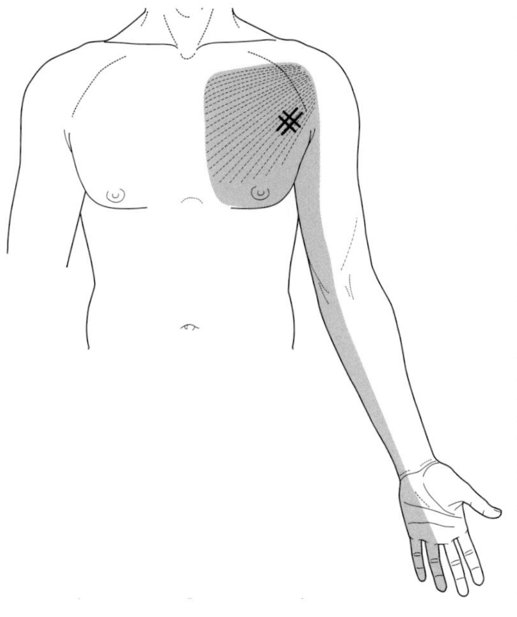

Figure 7.2 Myofascial trigger point in pectoralis major referring pain to chest and arm.

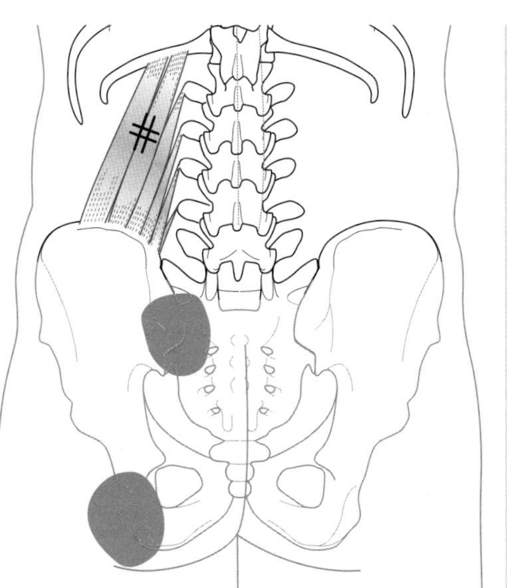

Figure 7.3 Myofascial trigger point in quadratus lumborum referring pain to sacrum and buttock.

Myofascial pain of gradual onset is likely to be caused by chronic, cumulative strain. This is common, for example, in the trapezius when many hours are spent in a poor working posture. A postural abnormality, such as kyphosis or scoliosis, puts extra strain on the muscles of the trunk (e.g. quadratus lumborum) or neck (e.g. trapezius). Constant mental tension can also produce prolonged muscle contraction: for example, tightly hunched shoulders may cause MTrPs to develop in the neck muscles, particularly trapezius.

Very occasionally, direct injury to the muscle can give rise to an MTrP, for example when it is compressed for a long period (e.g. sitting in a chair where the front edge compresses the hamstrings).

Because of the way MTrPs are caused by injury, they are often unilateral, though this is not always obvious in those that develop in the spinal muscles.

Primary MTrPs are usually unilateral.

Other causes of myofascial trigger points

MTrPs can develop in painful conditions, and then cause added problems for the patient. This is referred to as secondary myofascial pain. For example, arthritis of the hip is associated with MTrPs in the gluteal muscles, and MTrPs may develop in pectoralis major after myocardial infarction. This can lead to a confusing clinical picture as two diagnoses can be implicated for one set of symptoms. It is important to diagnose the original condition and give definitive treatment, but it may also be helpful to treat the MTrPs.

There is a strong relationship between the abdominal viscera and the muscles of the abdominal wall, via the nervous system. MTrPs can develop in the abdominal muscle wall after an acute condition, such as gastroenteritis, and subsequently cause pain and other symptoms, such as diarrhoea, even though the original condition has settled.

The diagnosis of an MTrP is not complete until an underlying cause is identified (whether injury or other condition).

Whenever pain occurs, including serious conditions such as cancer, an MTrP may also occur and confuse the diagnosis. Therefore, we cannot overemphasize the importance of making a conventional diagnosis.

Precipitating and perpetuating factors

Sometimes, the history of injury appears to be too trivial to have produced an MTrP, in which case the muscles may have been in a particularly vulnerable state. This can happen for a variety of reasons:

- Emotional: stress and anxiety, excitement
- Physical: exhaustion, poor muscle fitness from lack of exercise or exposure to cold
- Metabolic: poor nutritional status, low vitamin levels, hypothyroidism or chronic infection.

These factors that precipitate an MTrP also perpetuate it, and will also interfere with the response to treatment. They may need to be corrected before treatment can be successful and lasting.

Emotional, physical or metabolic factors can perpetuate an MTrP.

Mechanism

An MTrP is best regarded as a pathophysiological disorder rather than a purely pathological one, so 'mechanism' is a more appropriate term than 'pathology'. An MTrP feels distinctly hard, and it is surprising that microscopy of biopsy specimens shows little more than increased spacing between the fibres, a little leukocyte infiltration, and some contraction of individual sarcomeres.

Most research on the mechanisms of MTrPs has concentrated on the muscle fibres rather than the overlying fascia, and that is the approach that we reflect here. However, it is important to keep in mind that MTrPs may involve the fascia and the name 'myofascial' was originally introduced because the pain was produced by stimulation of the fascia, as well as the muscle.

Electrical activity has been detected from electromyography (EMG) needles placed within 1 mm of an MTrP (Hubbard & Berkoff 1993). This activity arises in muscle endplates, and is called 'miniature endplate potentials' (MEPPs). It shows the effect of the release of packets of acetylcholine (ACh) in an abnormal fashion. It is this persistent release of ACh that is the basic marker of an MTrP. Simons (Mense & Simons 1999) has proposed a hypothesis (Fig. 7.4) in which trauma to the endplate sets off the following sequence:

- Sustained release of ACh
- Inhibition of calcium pump
- Endplate depolarizes in an uncoordinated way, the potential is not propagated along the muscle cell wall
- Local contracture of sarcomeres in the immediate vicinity of the endplates
- Muscle shortening.

Although this is still a hypothesis and not yet an established mechanism, one of the predictions that arise from it has been supported in further experimentation: there is an accumulation of nociceptive transmitters around an MTrP (Shah et al 2005).

Clinical features

Presenting symptoms

Patients with active MTrPs usually present with a deep ache or pain. More rarely, they present with the associated stiffness or restriction of movement. Symptoms can vary greatly in severity – both between different patients, and over time in the same patient – often for no obvious reason.

MTrP pain is usually deep and aching, and fluctuates for no apparent reason.

The pain is usually referred away from the MTrP, and the painful zone may not even include the MTrP itself. For example, trapezius refers pain to the

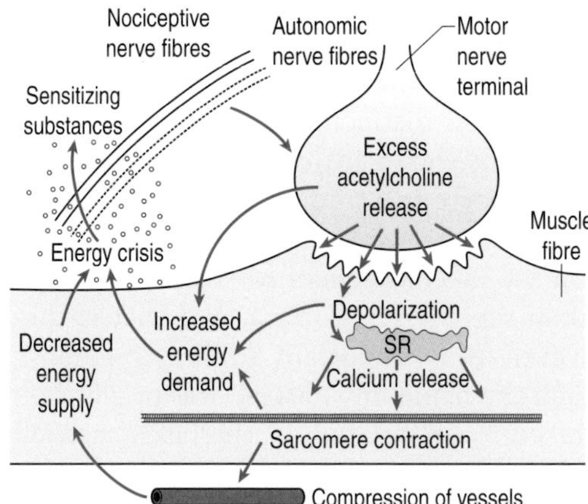

Figure 7.4 Integrated hypothesis of mechanism of myofascial trigger point. The primary dysfunction hypothesized here is an abnormal increase (by several orders of magnitude) in the production and release of acetylcholine packets from the motor nerve terminal under resting conditions. The greatly increased number of miniature endplate potentials (MEPPs) produces endplate noise and sustained depolarization of the postjunctional membrane of the muscle fibre. This sustained depolarization could cause a continuous release and inadequate uptake of calcium ions from local sarcoplasmic reticulum (SR) and produce sustained shortening (contracture) of sarcomeres. Each of these four highlighted changes would increase energy demand. The sustained muscle fibre shortening compresses local blood vessels, thereby reducing the nutrient and oxygen supplies that normally meet the energy demands of this region. The increased energy demand in the face of an impaired energy supply would produce a local energy crisis, which leads to release of sensitizing substances that could interact with autonomic and sensory (some nociceptive) nerves traversing that region. Subsequent release of neuroactive substances could, in turn, contribute to excessive acetylcholine release from the nerve terminal, completing what then becomes a self-sustaining vicious cycle. (Reproduced with permission from Simons D G, Travell J G, Simons L S 1999 Travell and Simons' Myofascial pain and dysfunction: the trigger point manual. Volume 1. Upper half of body. 2nd edn. Williams & Wilkins, Baltimore.)

neck and head, and there may be little pain at the site of the MTrP. The pain referral pattern for each muscle is reasonably consistent, so an accurate description is important in identifying the MTrP (Simons et al 1999, Travell & Simons 1983).

The patterns are often reminiscent of the 'channels' of traditional Chinese acupuncture, and they may well be the same phenomenon (Hong 2000). For example, the MTrP in trapezius is at the location of GB21, and the pain referral zone is remarkably similar to the Gall bladder channel as shown in Figure 7.5.

The pain pattern may reveal the location of the MTrP.

Patients with very active MTrPs show a characteristic clinical picture: the pain is deep, gripping and unremitting; the patient is restless, continually

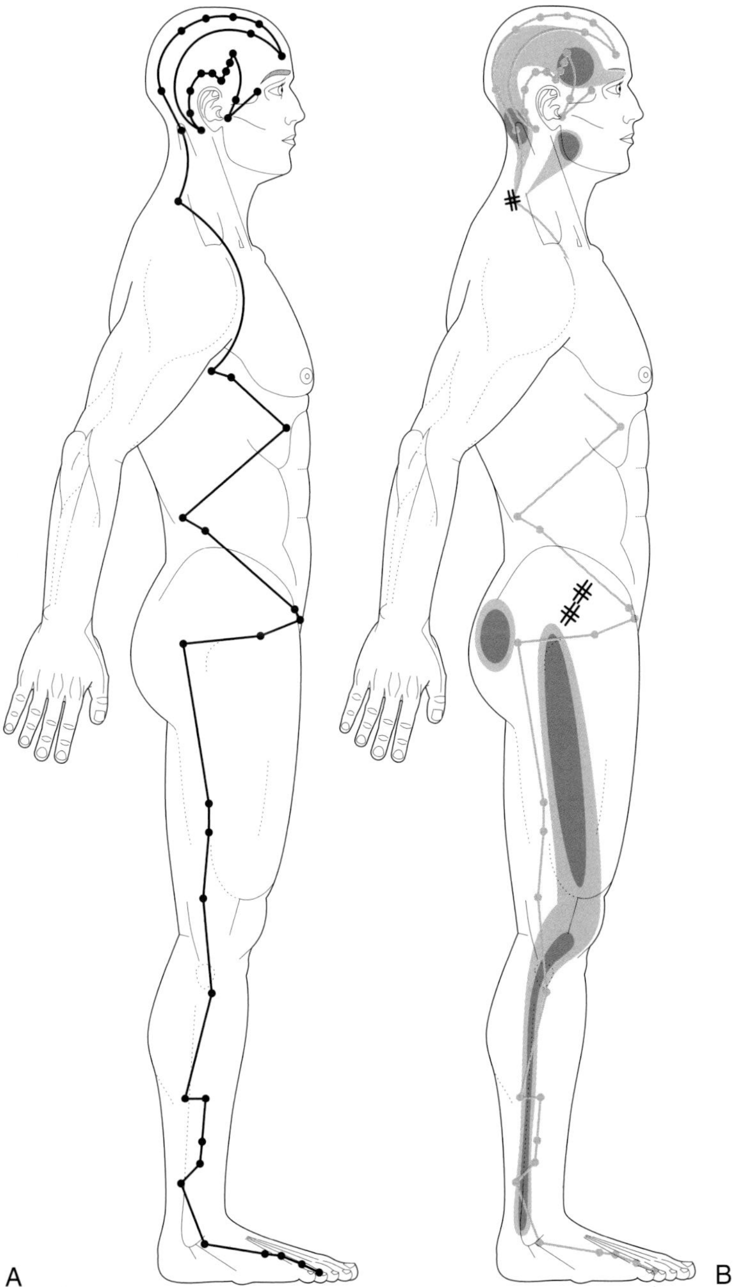

Figure 7.5 The correlation between trigger points and acupuncture points. (A) The trigger point in the upper fibres of trapezius is equivalent to the classical point GB21, and refers pain around the neck and head in a way that is remarkably similar to the GB meridian. (B) The trigger points in gluteus minimus are close to GB30 and GB31 (allowing for variation due to the patient's position) and refer pain down the leg to the ankle, in a pattern which is very close to the classical description of the GB meridian.

pressing deep and hard in the painful area, or stretching the affected part to try to relieve the pain. Movement may ease the pain and patients may even walk the streets at night in an attempt to escape the pain. If the patient can get rest in bed, the pain may be set off again if the muscle is kept shortened. For example, a patient with an MTrP in the left pectoralis major who sleeps on their side with the left arm folded across the chest is likely to wake in pain from the shortened muscle. Patients might sit or lie in an unnatural posture to keep the muscle in a lengthened position – the 'position of ease'. Patients often try to relieve the pain with a hot shower or bath.

The pain from an acute MTrP may simulate a medical or surgical emergency.

Less active MTrPs produce a less dramatic clinical picture: the pain and stiffness seem similar in many ways to the picture of osteoarthritis – which often co-exists. The pain is often deep and aching in nature, and the stiffness is worst after immobilization and eases with exercise.

History: direct questioning

It is important to obtain a precise history of the injury in cases of sudden onset, and details of work pattern in cases of insidious onset. Aggravating and relieving factors may help in establishing which muscle contains the MTrP. Pain due to MTrPs is often worse in cold weather, at times of stress and anxiety and, anecdotally, just before or during menstruation.

A few MTrPs have pathognomonic symptoms, such as the superficial prickling sensations over the chin and face from MTrPs in the platysma. Interested practitioners can discover these with experience, as long as they keep an open mind about the cause of 'peculiar' symptoms, and keep a copy of a detailed reference book close at hand, such as Travell and Simons' manual.

History: other symptoms

Occasionally, autonomic symptoms dominate the clinical picture: for example, one MTrP in the sternomastoid muscle causes dizziness and disorientation rather than pain.

The shortening and swelling of some muscles leads to pressure on nearby nerves and produces symptoms of nerve entrapment. For example, an MTrP in the piriformis can compress the sciatic nerve as it passes through the greater sciatic foramen. The patient may complain not only of the pain in a typical referral pattern, but also of paraesthesiae and numbness in the leg, as shown in Figure 7.6. This combination of symptoms is easily confused with sciatica caused by nerve-root compression.

Trigger points and spinal pain

MTrPs commonly cause spinal pain, or at least contribute to it. Low back pain may be produced by MTrPs in muscles of the various paravertebral groups (multifidi, longitudinal group, additional muscles such as quadratus

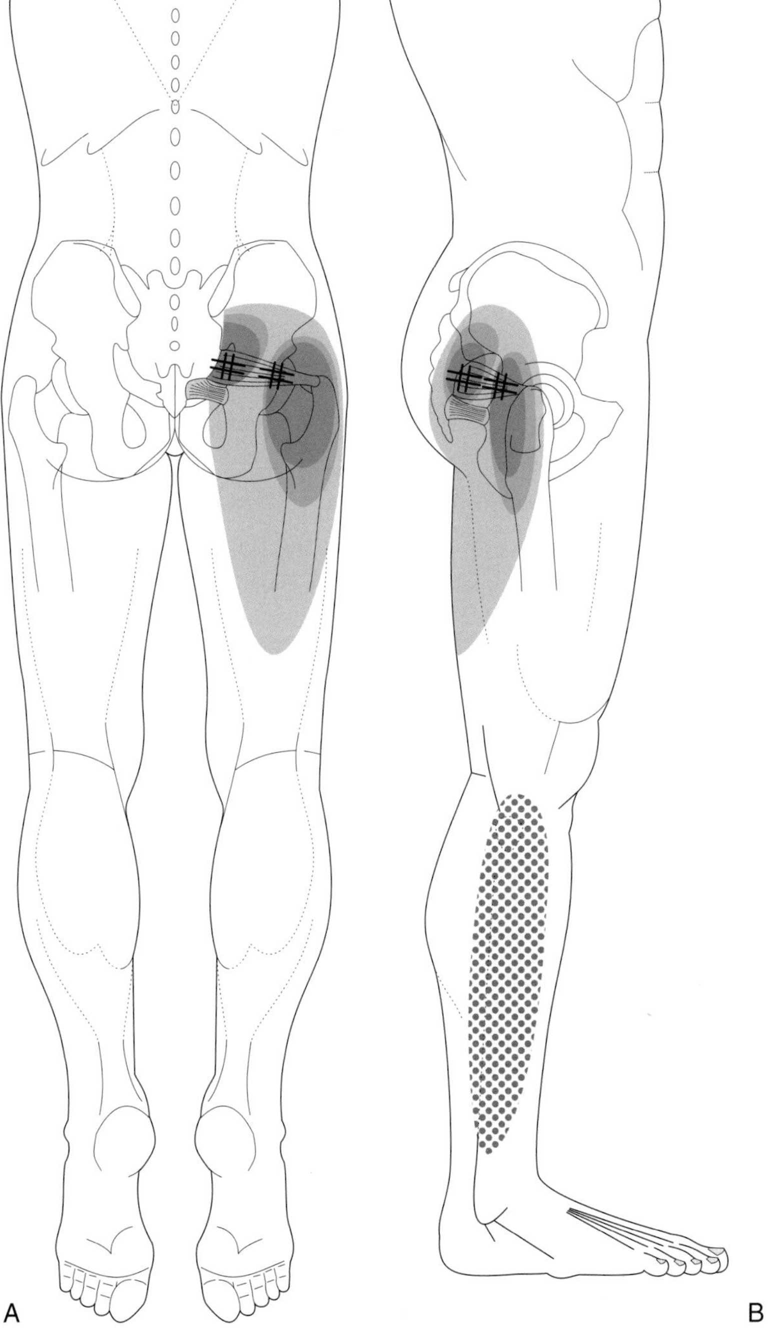

Figure 7.6 This figure shows trigger points in the (A) medial and (B) lateral sections of the piriformis muscle, which can lead to shortening of the muscle. This shortening compresses the sciatic nerve causing paraesthesiae in the lower leg. The important point to note is that paraesthesiae in the leg are not invariably caused by lesions to the nerve root.

lumborum) or the hip girdle such as piriformis. Neck pain may be due to MTrPs in the neck muscles, or in the shoulder girdle muscles, such as trapezius. Patients who have been told their X-ray films show 'degenerative change' may actually have pain that is due to MTrPs.

MTrPs may mimic other medical conditions.

Diagnosis

A convincing diagnosis of an MTrP can be made when the following features are found on history and examination:

- A history of pain that fluctuates for no good reason
- A taut band in the muscle
- An area of tenderness in the taut band
- Patient's pain reproduced by pressure on the tender area
- Passive stretch of the muscle restricted by pain.

Proper examination for MTrPs requires a good knowledge of anatomy, and many acupuncturists find they need to re-learn the attachments and functions of muscle.

Palpation

It is important to be able to identify an MTrP by palpation, to make the diagnosis and needle it precisely. It is crucially important to draw the fingers *across* the muscle, at right angles to the fibres. Many clinicians are used to feeling through muscles to the structure below: this is one of the rare occasions when it is the muscle fibres themselves that are of interest.

Firstly, prepare and position the patient so that the muscle is:

- not tense – the patient has to be warm, relaxed and comfortable, with the part well supported. This usually involves treating the patient lying down, with pillows for support
- accessible – a limb might have to be placed in a particular position; for example, pectoralis major in the anterior axillary wall can only be examined fully with the arm abducted; quadratus lumborum can only be accessed with the patient lying on the opposite side, with the upper leg lowered right on to the couch to open the angle between the ribs and the iliac crest
- the right length – if the fibres are fully stretched the taut band may not be palpable, if fully shortened the bulk of the muscle hides the MTrP. The appropriate length is achieved by moving the limb, for example increasing or decreasing the abduction of the arm when examining pectoralis major.

Examine for MTrPs by drawing the fingers across the muscle fibres.

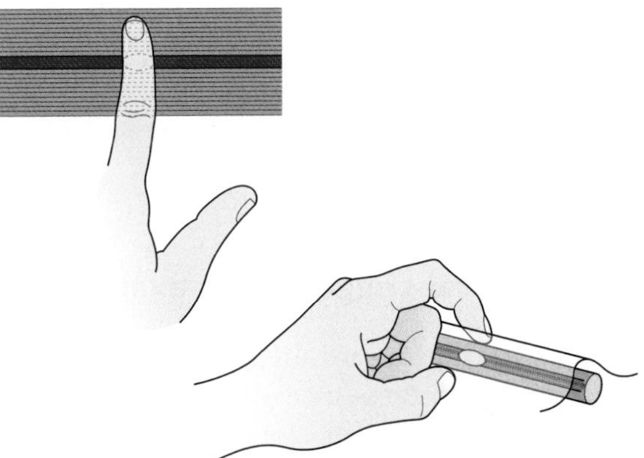

Figure 7.7 Diagrams showing flat palpation of myofascial trigger points and pincer palpation when the muscle belly can be encircled with the fingers.

There are two techniques for palpation: flat or pincer (see Fig. 7.7). In both cases the fingers are drawn across the fibres. Flat palpation is suitable for most muscles, such as quadratus lumborum or the medial portion of pectoralis major. But if part of the muscle can be lifted off underlying structures – for example, the upper trapezius, the lateral portion of pectoralis major in the anterior axillary fold, or the teres major and latissimus dorsi in the posterior axillary fold – the examiner's fingers and thumb encircle the muscle, and gently and systematically palpate it between the tip of a finger and the tip of the thumb. It does not take long to learn to recognize normal muscle fibre density and to identify the thicker, harder 'taut band', like a rope running the length of the muscle.

Having identified the band, then examine it gently for a tender spot, which is the MTrP itself, usually at about the midpoint. Finally, press on the tender spot for about 5 seconds and ask the patient what he or she feels. The best response is: 'That's my pain', i.e. pain recognition. Be careful not to hint that that is the response you want, as some patients will be eager to please you. The patient's pain is also likely to be reproduced by needling.

Forceful examination can aggravate MTrPs.

Twitch response

Trigger points may show another clinical sign on palpation – the twitch response – but remember that this may be painful and is not necessary for diagnosis. It is produced by 'snapping' palpation, which involves a firmer pull or tweak across the fibres, rather like twanging a guitar string in slow motion. It appears as a brief twitch under the skin, in line with the MTrP. It does not involve the whole muscle, like a tendon reflex, and should be distinguished from the effect of simply snapping the muscle border. Twitch responses should be generated during treatment with the needle, since they are regarded as a sign that treatment is likely to be effective.

A twitch response, with pain recognition, from needling is likely to indicate a favourable outcome.

Difficulties in myofascial trigger point examination

Palpation is not always straightforward. In deeper muscles, such as piriformis, the MTrP is not accessible. In these cases, a careful history is important, and examination for limitation of range of movement and weakness. In addition, compare the two sides: MTrPs are generally unilateral, at least in the early stages. Accurate palpation is difficult in patients who are obese.

MTrP pain is usually limited to one side (or the midline).

Patients rarely have a single MTrP; other nearby muscles are also likely to develop MTrPs. It is important to note that both the target area and the trigger point may be tender: only the MTrP has the taut band, tender nodule and pain recognition on pressure. When practitioners first start examining muscles, they often find difficulty in distinguishing between tender points (there are often many) and MTrPs (there are usually few). The key to success is to concentrate on developing the feel for a taut band. Diagnosis becomes easier with experience and practice, but sometimes it is simply not possible to be sure if a particular tender point is the origin of the pain. In this case, it is entirely justifiable to treat the point speculatively, but carefully, as a 'therapeutic trial'.

Tenderness of the pain reference zone can be a distraction: the MTrP itself must be found.

Differential diagnosis

Suspect an MTrP if the clinical picture suggests a musculoskeletal condition (i.e. is related to activity), but does not precisely match another clinical diagnosis. Anomalous symptoms that are often labelled 'atypical' or 'idiopathic' could be due to MTrPs, for example atypical facial pain. Several conditions may give rise to MTrP pain that persists and may cause difficulty in diagnosing a chronic problem, as shown in Table 7.1.

Investigations

There are no investigations that can assist the diagnosis of MTrPs. Thermography has been suggested, but subsequently rejected as unreliable. Ultrasound and MRI have not, up to now, revealed any diagnostic features. Electromyography may be diagnostic, but is only relevant as a research tool. Blood tests are

TABLE 7.1

Myofascial trigger points that develop secondary to medical conditions and produce a similar clinical picture

Original condition	Persistent functional diagnosis	Muscles typically involved	Somatovisceral symptoms
Myocardial infarction	Post-infarction pain	Pectoralis major	Chest pain
Oesophagitis	Chronic epigastric pain	Rectus abdominis	Epigastric burning pain, nausea, anorexia, vomiting
Gastroenteritis	Irritable bowel syndrome	Rectus abdominis, internal obliques and external obliques	Pain, diarrhoea, constipation, bloating
Cystitis	Chronic cystitis	Lower rectus abdominis	Lower abdominal pain and frequency of micturition
Dysmenorrhoea	Chronic pelvic pain	Lower rectus abdominis	Cramping lower abdominal and pelvic pain

of no value, except that they may be useful to exclude hypothyroidism if this is clinically suspected, because it may cause resistance to treatment.

Treatment techniques

Needling is not the only way to treat MTrPs, but it is quick and effective. This section is not intended on its own to give enough information to guide treatment with needles: full details of needling techniques are given in Chapter 12. There are four general approaches to needling MTrPs:

1. Direct deep needling, which means inserting the needle directly into the MTrP itself. This is swift and effective for acute MTrPs. The practitioner must know the local anatomy to avoid serious harm. Very often the MTrP is not located on the first thrust of the needle, and repeated thrusts are needed, spreading in a fan-like pattern from the skin insertion point (called 'fan-like lift and thrust') (Fig. 12.2). Direct needling seems to have a local effect, but it is not clear precisely what that is: it may simply physically disrupt the dysfunctional unit, and perhaps provoke local vasodilation, which assists tissue healing.
2. Superficial needling, which is simply inserting the needle into the tissues precisely over the site of the MTrP. When using this method, it is essential that all tender MTrPs are treated together in the treatment session, and that treatment is repeated until they are no longer tender.

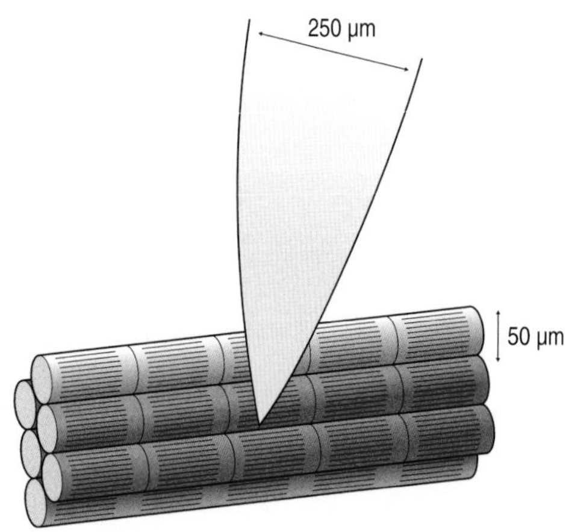

Figure 7.8 Tip of acupuncture needle in relation to skeletal muscle fibres, drawn to scale.

The mechanism of this effect is unknown, and not based on obvious anatomical connections since the overlying skin usually has different innervation from the MTrP. It is very acceptable to patients, and unlikely to cause reactions. It is particularly useful for treating MTrPs situated in an anatomical area where deep needling carries excess risk, for example in the anterior neck or just medial to the scapula.

3. Needling local classical Chinese acupuncture points seems to have some effect on MTrPs, from clinical observation.
4. Electroacupuncture (see Chapter 12) is mainly used to treat chronic MTrPs. Insert one needle into the MTrP, the other a few centimetres away along the MTrP band.

After needling MTrPs, ask the patient to move the affected part through its full range of movement, slowly and deliberately, to achieve a gentle stretch. This helps to inactivate the MTrP and re-educate both the muscle and its owner that the muscle shortening has been abolished and the range of movement is normal. At the same time, warn patients not to overload the muscle.

After needling, stretch the muscle slowly – but do not overload it.

Patients should also be warned that they may feel soreness in the muscle for a few hours after treatment, and can use a hot-water bottle, bath, shower or their usual analgesic medication for relief. Simple analgesics seem more effective than non-steroidal anti-inflammatory drugs.

These recommendations on needling are based on clinical experience, since there is little definitive research on treatment techniques. Some practitioners, particularly in America, inject MTrPs with local anaesthetic, saline, steroid solution or botulinum toxin, but a systematic review found none of these was superior to dry needling (Cummings & White 2001). Botulinum toxin has a theoretical advantage since it blocks release of acetylcholine and thus may 'switch off' the pathological mechanism of the MTrP at source, but early studies have been disappointing. Other physical therapies that are likely to work for MTrPs include deep massage and stretch of various sorts.

Prognosis

MTrPs of recent onset, limited to a single muscle and not overly active, may respond very swiftly to needling, possibly even to a single treatment. However, when MTrPs have developed in several muscles in a group and have been present for more than about 6 months, treatment needs to be repeated weekly for several weeks and patients may need to work hard at active stretching exercises between treatments to reinforce the effect of needling. Even so, the MTrP may not dissipate permanently, but revert to being a latent MTrP.

A patient can reduce the likelihood of reactivating latent MTrPs by continuing a daily stretching routine, keeping the muscle warm, and avoiding overload, which includes correcting underlying ergonomic or postural stresses.

It is interesting to note that some patients who have had successful MTrP therapy feel a major improvement in their general wellbeing. The physical limitation, pain and the sleep disturbance caused by the MTrP had adverse effects on their lives in ways that they had not recognized until they were treated. This fact may contribute to the improvement in wellbeing that is frequently reported as a general benefit after acupuncture treatment.

Summary

MTrPs arise when a muscle or its associated fascia fail to heal after injury, and should be distinguished from other tender points. MTrP pain is probably under-diagnosed through lack of awareness of the condition. Sufficient clinical and scientific evidence has accumulated for it to be considered in a differential diagnosis.

The cause of MTrPs is usually acute injury or chronic cumulative strain from postural problems or repetitive activity. They may also arise in other painful conditions, for example in the abdominal muscles from referred visceral pain. They occur at relatively fixed positions in each muscle.

Certain factors precipitate and perpetuate MTrPs, including strong emotions, physical states such as exhaustion, and certain metabolic conditions, including hypothyroidism.

One hypothesis for the mechanism of MTrPs involves sustained release of acetylcholine at the muscle endplate and sustained contraction of individual sarcomeres. This creates additional energy demands, but impedes circulation, thus perpetuating the problem and releasing nociceptive transmitters.

Patients with MTrPs usually present because of the pain. The trigger point may vary in activity from acutely painful, through chronic persistent pain to latent, i.e. only causing stiffness. The pattern of pain is typical for each individual trigger point and may assist in finding the point. MTrPs commonly contribute to the overall picture of spinal pain, whether or not other pathology is present. MTrPs frequently cause symptoms that mimic other conditions. The predominant clinical features of MTrPs are the palpable taut band, tender point and patient recognition of pain.

Treatment with acupuncture usually involves deep, precise needling of the MTrP, though some recommend superficial needling. Electroacupuncture is sometimes used for chronic cases, although this is the one circumstance where vigorous manual needling may be more effective if tolerated by the patient. The patient should put the affected muscle(s) through a complete range of movement after needling. The prognosis is good, provided the MTrP is treated early and perpetuating factors can be removed. Chronic MTrPs may be successfully inactivated with repeated treatment, but are less likely to be abolished permanently.

Further reading

Baldry P E 2005 Acupuncture, trigger points and musculoskeletal pain. 3rd edn. Elsevier, Edinburgh

This text provides a thorough explanation of the most common myofascial trigger points encountered in practice. The author recommends treatment by superficial needling.

Simons D G, Travell J G, Simons L S 1999 The trigger point manual. 2nd edn. Williams & Wilkins, Baltimore

This pair of books is expensive, but regarded as the canon of myofascial trigger points pain. Full of terrific detail and wonderful anatomical diagrams to serve as a handbook for life time of practice.

CHAPTER

8

Traditional Chinese acupuncture reinterpreted

Contents

After reading this chapter you should be able to:

- outline the origins and background of traditional Chinese acupuncture
- discuss some traditional concepts and their limitations
- describe why a radical reappraisal is now needed.

Introduction

The last five chapters have described approaches to acupuncture that are consistent with current views of the body. Why do we now describe the traditional views? Partly because we want to add to the discussion on how acupuncture in traditional Chinese medicine (TCM) may have developed in the first place, partly because we believe patients should be aware of the basis of the acupuncture treatment given by a TCA practitioner, and partly because we think there may be aspects of TCA that still have something to offer.

'Acupuncture' (literally, acus = needle + pungere to puncture or prick, from the Latin) is a European word that is an attempt to represent the

Chinese 'zhen-jiu', which means 'needle and moxa' therapy (Birch & Kaptchuk 1999, Lu & Needham 1980, Schnorrenberger 2003). TCA deserves the respect due to any therapy that has such a long history of a consistent, structured, and academic approach. Acupuncture and traditional Chinese herbal medicine remain the treatment of choice for some populations, at least for some conditions.

But there is a difference between respect and unquestioning acceptance. TCM is still taught and practised using models and methods that have not been updated in the light of scientific discoveries, in the way that Hippocratic medicine has. We think that is a problem and a weakness. As we shall see, the approach to acupuncture was continually updated for centuries in the light of new information about the structure and function of the body. Why should that process stop now? We believe Western medical acupuncture is simply the latest chapter in an evolving story.

While the Chinese theories of acupuncture may be attractive and 'real' in the sense of apparently explaining symptoms, they often appear outdated and even incorrect to someone trained in health care in the scientific era. Learning TCA involves suspending one's natural critical appraisal, which someone who is trained in health care is unlikely to want to do. This chapter, which is unavoidably superficial, attempts to describe some of the concepts of TCM and to point out some of its deficiencies; it is very much a personal view.

Chinese origins of acupuncture

The idea that acupuncture originated in China about 2000 years ago is widely accepted. However, it may be only partially correct, as we discuss below.

The first known text on acupuncture is the Huang Di Nei Jing *The Yellow Emperor's Internal Classic* (Veith 1949), which is said to date from 200–100 BC. This detailed work describes systems of diagnosis and treatment with herbs and needles, though does not name acupuncture points. The text of the *Yellow Emperor's Internal Classic* is likely to be a compilation of traditions that had evolved over preceding years (Kaplan 1997). The information is presented in the form of questions posed by the Emperor and answered by his minister, Chhi-Po. Medical problems are discussed in terms of the Taoist world view, which was prevalent at the time. This text is regarded as the founding canon of Chinese medicine, rather in the way that Hippocrates' works were the foundation of Western medicine (Kaptchuk 1983). However, unlike Hippocrates, the text is still used as treatment guidelines.

Modern readers find it difficult to embrace the full meaning of the text because of the remoteness of culture and concepts. Often an intuitive explanation turns out to be quite wrong: for example, the meridians could be thought of as lines connecting acupuncture points: however, the meridians came first, as documents found in a burial tomb dating from 168 BC refer to a system of meridians, but not points (Chen 1997).

European origins of acupuncture

Prehistoric human remains have produced tantalizing evidence that acupuncture may have originated in Europe. Ötzi the 'Tyrolean Ice Man' was a hunter whose body was preserved in an Alpine glacier in about 3300 BC, emerging from the melting face in 1991 (Dorfer et al 1998). Ötzi's body carries 47 tattoo marks, organized in 15 groups, mainly on the back and legs (Plates 6A and B). The tattoos consist of spots or lines of charcoal deposited in the subcutaneous layer of the skin. Because they are situated in areas that would be covered in clothes, and because of their shape, these tattoos do not seem to have the same purpose as most tattoos from that era – decoration or ritual. Instead, it has been suggested that they have some medical purpose, and may be signs of cautery, which is a common feature of folk medicine (Nogier 1981).

Dorfer was interested in Ötzi's tattoos, and was inspired to consult some acupuncture experts about them (Dorfer et al 1999). After careful measurements, these experts concluded that nine of the 15 groups of tattoos lie within a few millimetres of classical acupuncture points. Even more suggestively, their locations are the same as the points that traditional Chinese acupuncturists might have used to treat the medical conditions that X-ray film and other examinations showed Ötzi to have had at the time he died:

- Bladder meridian points on the back and the leg for spinal degeneration
- LR8, SP6 and GB points for an intestinal problem – infestation with worms.

Ötzi's tattoos, therefore, suggest that a system of treatment that was remarkably similar to Chinese acupuncture existed in Europe long before any evidence of it in China. While this interpretation is speculative, it challenges the idea that the Chinese had a monopoly on acupuncture.

The evolution of acupuncture in China

Acupuncture continued to evolve over the centuries that followed its description in the *Yellow Emperor's Internal Classic*, and in some areas it was regarded as routine therapy together with herbs, massage, diet and moxibustion (heat). About the end of the first millennium, Wang Wei-Yi (987–1067) constructed hollow bronze statues (Plate 7) that clearly depicted acupuncture points as holes (Ma 1992). During the Ming Dynasty (1368–1644), *The Great Compendium of Acupuncture and Moxibustion* was published, giving clear descriptions of 361 points that form the basis of modern acupuncture.

Acupuncture was not practised everywhere in China, and the approach to treatment was far from uniform throughout the country (Birch & Kaptchuk 1999). Many different esoteric theories of diagnosis and treatment emerged, sometimes even contradicting each other, largely due to vast distances between centres and lack of communication that resulted in local traditions. Rival acupuncture schools tried to establish their exclusiveness and influence.

Interest in acupuncture declined from the 17th century onwards as it came to be regarded as superstitious and irrational in comparison to Western medicine (Baldry 1993, Ma 1992). Acupuncture was finally excluded from the Imperial Medical Institute by decree of the Emperor in 1822. The knowledge and skill were retained, however, both as an interest among academics and as a therapy among rural healers. The final ignominy for acupuncture arrived in 1929 when it was outlawed, along with other forms of TCM (Ma 1992).

After the installation of the Communist government in 1949, traditional forms of medicine, including acupuncture, were reinstated, possibly both out of national pride and sheer practicality: low-cost medicine was the only means of providing even basic levels of health care to the massive population. Mao Tse-tung promoted TCM with the words, 'Let a thousand flowers flourish' – though it is reported that Mao himself rejected acupuncture for his illnesses and used Western medicine (Basser 1999).

During this renaissance of traditional healing, an attempt was made to form a consensus of all the divergent strands of herbal medicine, acupuncture and moxibustion, and to produce a unified version of TCM (Birch & Kaptchuk 1999). TCM became available in Western-style hospitals in China, though not in the same departments as Western medicine. At about the same time, acupuncture research institutes were established and several researchers in China sought more rational explanations of acupuncture, such as Ji-Sheng Han in Beijing who undertook ground-breaking research on the release of neurotransmitters (Han & Terenius 1982).

The worldwide spread of acupuncture

Through China's influence on its neighbours, Korea and Japan assimilated acupuncture and herbal medicine around the 6th century (Baldry 1993) and both countries still use these therapies, often in parallel with Western medicine. Acupuncture arrived in Vietnam when commercial routes opened up in the 8th to 10th centuries. In the West, France was one of the first countries to adopt acupuncture (Kaplan 1997). Reports of acupuncture were brought back by Jesuit missionaries from the 16th century onwards, and the practice was embraced by some French clinicians. Berlioz, father of the composer, ran clinical trials on acupuncture and wrote papers on it in 1816 (Bivens 2000). The French style of acupuncture was deeply influenced by a diplomat, Soulier de Morant, who spent many years in China and published a number of treatises on the subject of acupuncture from 1939 onwards.

Willem Ten Rhijne was the first Western doctor to write a description of acupuncture, in about 1680. He was a physician to the East India Company and witnessed acupuncture practice in Japan (Bivens 2000). Much later, in the first half of the 19th century, there was a flurry of interest in America and Britain, and a number of publications appeared in the scientific literature including an editorial article in the Lancet entitled 'acupuncturation' (Anon. 1823). But by the middle of the 19th century, acupuncture was no longer of interest, though it was briefly resurrected in one edition of Sir William

Osler's textbook of medicine (Osler 1912). He suggested that acupuncture was the best treatment for acute lumbago, and any needle would do, even a lady's hat-pin!

The 20th century

In 1971, James Reston, a senior reporter for *The New York Times*, was visiting China in preparation for President Nixon's visit. He required emergency surgery for appendicitis, and during the recovery period he developed paralytic ileus, which was treated with acupuncture. He described the experience in his influential column (Reston 1971) and subsequently several teams of US physicians made fact-finding tours of China to assess acupuncture. They were particularly interested in its use for surgical analgesia, though they eventually concluded that acupuncture was not reliable as a sole analgesic. Their reports stimulated a number of research studies, particularly in treating experimental pain in volunteers. Acupuncture finally gained a certain amount of respectability in the USA after the positive conclusions of a NIH consensus conference (NIH Consensus Development Panel 1998).

Individual doctors from the UK also visited China to see acupuncture for themselves, and made a persistent effort to reconsider the traditional explanations of acupuncture in scientific terms (Baldry 2005a), as discussed in the Introduction.

We shall now briefly describe a selection of the traditional concepts and speculate on how they might have arisen.

Traditional Chinese acupuncture theories

The context of traditional Chinese acupuncture

Acupuncture was practised in China as part of medicine, together with herbs, massage and dietary manipulation. Presumably Chinese doctors had to deal with the typical major diseases common to any early civilization, including major infections such as tuberculosis, acute sepsis, meningitis and abscesses; congenital disorders and deformities; chronic conditions such as heart failure or hyper- and hypothyroidism; trauma and fractures; as well as acute surgical emergencies. Strong and invasive treatments were developed, and it is interesting to compare early medicine in the West, which used drastic treatments such as blood-letting and purgation. The arrival of active pharmaceuticals, particularly antibiotics, changed the face of medicine.

There is no single theory of traditional acupuncture, and even the attempt in the 1950s to unify it into TCM fails to satisfy all practitioners. It seems that some physicians would just treat symptoms and signs, but others also wanted to know about the constitution of the individual as a prerequisite (Kaptchuk 1983). They would take into account the patient's preferences for one kind of weather or another, the colour of their skin, their favourite foods, or the time of year of the onset of symptoms. Disease was seen as an integral and perhaps inevitable part of a person's very existence, rather than a condition produced by a single identifiable cause.

Chinese approaches to acupuncture use various combinations of the following basic concepts.

Chinese anatomy and physiology

It is important to credit the ancient Chinese physicians with some remarkable discoveries; their understanding of the structure and function of the body was an impressive achievement for its day, well in advance of Western anatomy and physiology at the time. They provided some great insights, such as the central importance of the liver for body metabolism and (probably) the concept of circulation of the blood. However, China was largely isolated from the scientific revolution in Europe, so the impact of the scientific understanding of anatomy and physiology on TCM was very limited (Kendall 2002).

Briefly, the Chinese considered that human physiology consists of the interaction of three vital substances – *qi*, Blood and Body fluids. *Qi* is the most fundamental of these: humans were born with 'hereditary *qi*', which is stored in the Kidneys and maintained by food and air so that it could circulate to nourish and defend the body. When *qi* becomes 'pathological' – deficiency, stagnation, rebellion for example – then symptoms arise and disease follows. At the risk of oversimplifying, deficiency of *qi* means cold, under activity or weakness; stagnation is probably equivalent to muscle spasm; and rebellion is exemplified by vomiting. Blood is a 'highly condensed' form of *qi* and inseparable from it. Body fluids derive from food: pure fluids enter the body and the impure fluids are secreted via the urinary tract. Blood and Body fluids can have disturbances of their own, which must be diagnosed and corrected.

Throughout this description, one can perceive the efforts of intelligent minds working out a theoretical explanation for their careful observations of man in health and disease. It is tempting to speculate how the Chinese derived their particular explanations for the structure and function of the body, and we shall give just three examples:

1. In TCM, the internal organs are classified as either solid or hollow. Oddly, both Lung and Heart were regarded as solid. Could physicians have been misled by the solid appearance of these organs at *post-mortem* examination?
2. In TCM the Heart is regarded as the 'seat of the mind' (Shenmen). Did this reflect the observation that the heart races when we become excited or afraid? Was the heart assumed to be the seat of both the racing pulse and the excitement?
3. In TCM, the Spleen was involved in the absorption of food: food enters the stomach, and an explanation had to be found for how it combines with air, in the lungs. Was it assumed to pass along the most obvious route – through the Spleen and then through the diaphragm? Naturally the diaphragm had to be perforated – which is exactly how it was perceived in Western medicine before Harvey's time.

Traditional acupuncturists still think of the Spleen as being closely associated with the stomach and digestion, which is far from the truth as we know it. When challenged, they say they think of the Spleen as a 'function' rather than a physical organ: the function attributed to the Spleen is transportation of food and fluids. This idea, which seems odd to modern minds, becomes compounded when TCM says that a 'deficiency of the Spleen' causes peripheral oedema: and the deficiency arises from an invasion of Dampness (Maciocia 1989), for example from sitting on damp surfaces.

Qi

Qi (pronounced as 'chee' in cheese) is a term used in acupuncture with two rather different meanings:

- *Qi* includes the sense of activity, or the potential for action: it is the difference between life and death, between still and sparkling water. It is similar to what is understood in physics as kinetic, potential or metabolic energy. Humans are considered to be born with an allocation of *qi*, and to replenish it with food and air, so that the *qi* can be distributed throughout the body as 'nourishment' and 'defence'. Disease arises when *qi* is disturbed: this can be an excess, a deficiency, or a blockage. This seems a reasonable approach to describing what we would know as (1) the supply of tissue nutrients such as oxygen and glucose, and (2) tissue repair and various immune functions.
- *Qi* is also sometimes used in the abstract sense of the Life Force in 'energetic medicine'. This is probably a misunderstanding which we shall not discuss further here (Kendall 2002, Schnorrenberger 2003, Soulié de Morant 1957).

Yin/Yang 'balance'

Another fundamental concept in TCA is the balance of opposites, represented as *yin* and *yang*. The original meanings of these words are the dark and light sides of a hill: *yin* is dark, cold and inactive, whereas *yang* is bright, hot and active. Sick people are considered to have an imbalance of *yin* and *yang*, and treatment is designed to rebalance them.

This concept is similar to Claude Bernard's *milieu internal*, i.e. what we understand as homeostasis – though of course many centuries older. It is easy to find examples in medicine where physiology involves 'balance' and disease involves the loss of this balance, either as the cause or the effect: temperature regulation; autonomic control of skin blood flow; gastrointestinal motility; thyrotoxicosis and hypothyroidism; hyper- and hypocorticosteroid conditions. But that does not mean that every medical condition can be seen as a disturbance of balance: infectious diseases, cancer, degenerative diseases and fractures, for example, cannot be explained in this way.

We speculate that one original – and very sound – observation came to be applied as a general rule in every situation: *yin/yang* balance evolved to become the vital basis of good health. The Chinese seemed to excel in making general rules out of accurate observations, and we shall see other examples of this tendency.

Five phases (elements)

The concept of five 'phases' is very ancient: the word translated as 'phases' has no exact equivalent in English and is often translated as 'elements', though it is more elaborate than the four elements of Greek or medieval European medicine: Earth, Air, Fire and Water (Maciocia 1989). It has nothing to do with the 'elements' of the periodic table. The concept behind the five phases is complex: everything – whether physical object, animal or human being – was thought to comprise five phases in every aspect of its existence: Wood, Fire, Earth, Metal and Water. Each of the phases has corresponding features in every aspect of life: for example, the type of emotional character, colour, season, direction and flavour. Thus, Wood corresponds with anger, the colour green, spring, the East and sour flavour. Moreover, each phase is also linked to a pair of organs – Wood, for example, is linked with Liver and Gall Bladder. So an upset in any of the phases would cause disease in these particular organs, and could be influenced by needling the meridians of the same name.

Each phase predominates at a different period of the day in a fixed cycle. Each phase influences the other phases; stimulating the one immediately following and inhibiting the one following that (Fig. 8.1) (Lawson-Wood & Lawson-Wood 1973).

Because the concept of five phases is circular, and everything relates to everything else, a practitioner can always argue that one single fault somewhere in the system has produced all the subsequent faults: all conditions are explicable as extensions of one fundamental imbalance. This gives an impression of holism, but is unconvincing.

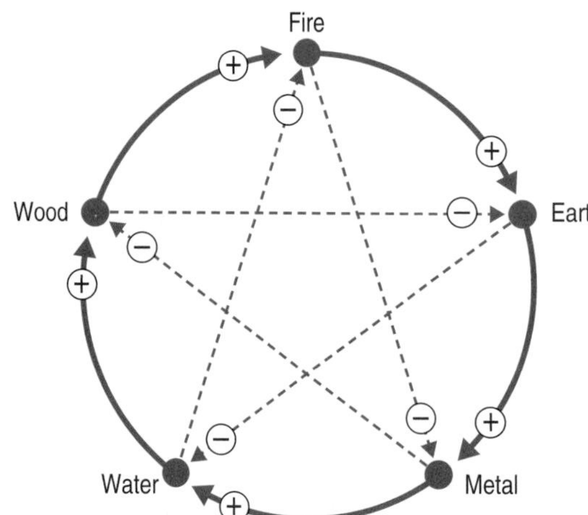

Figure 8.1 Diagram of the cycle of five phases, indicating interrelationships: each phase supposedly stimulates the next (e.g. Water, Wood) and inhibits the subsequent one (e.g. Water, Fire).

Meridians

The Chinese used the word *jing-luo* to describe a bundle of vessels, channels or *meridians*. Some authorities argue that these were palpable physical structures; almost certainly what we now know as blood vessels, nerves and tendons (Schnorrenberger 2003).

When the concept of fixed acupuncture points developed, there seems to have been a quite separate idea of meridians that were used as an *aide memoir* for finding them – rather as, in modern astronomy, the constellations are used to remember the position of the stars. Even if the stars themselves are unrelated, their position can be remembered from where they appear in relation to the other stars.

The concept of meridians was used in various ways in clinical practice:

- Diseases 'invaded' the meridian, i.e. superficial symptoms would lead to damage of the associated organ – unless they were repulsed by acupuncture
- Needling of the meridians would improve the condition of the associated organ
- In the five-phases approach, each meridian was supposed to have 'control points' that directly influenced the meridians of the other phases
- Points at the end of a meridian were needled to treat a painful condition elsewhere on the meridian.

Acupuncture points

We discussed the concepts of acupuncture points, and possible explanations of their origin, in Chapter 3.

Associated effect points

The Bladder meridians (one on each side of the body) run down alongside the spine and onwards down the back of the legs. As the meridians run about 4 cm from the midline, over the longitudinal muscles, classical points are shown at almost every spinal segmental level. Some of these have come to be associated with having an effect on one or other of the organs. Interestingly, the associated organ is innervated by that segmental level, as discussed under viscerotomes in Chapter 4 and shown in Figure 8.2. This illustrates that the Chinese approach to acupuncture does actually acknowledge biomedical concepts.

Diagnosis in traditional Chinese medicine

Tongue diagnosis

TCM practitioners may inspect the tongue carefully for its colouring and texture, looking at the margins of the tongue and the body. They use information

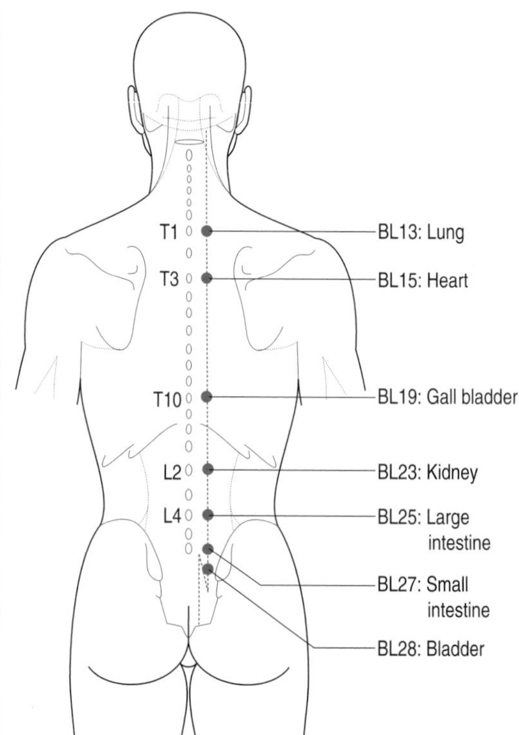

Figure 8.2 The 'associated effect points' of traditional Chinese acupuncture, demonstrating a biomedical understanding of the segmental innervation of the viscera.

from the tongue in forming a diagnosis. Now, some clinical conditions, such as severe iron-deficiency anaemia, acute Streptococcal infection, or local Candida infection, do show distinctive and even florid changes in the appearance of the tongue. It seems possible that these known associations in a few particular cases have been extended to make a general rule – that the tongue always provides information in making a diagnosis.

Pulse diagnosis

TCA practitioners often study the pulse in great detail, and claim to glean much more information from it than Western physicians do. Some say it gives information on the state of the meridians (e.g. Liver deficiency); others use a general description ('slippery' pulse). It is a common observation that some conditions do produce highly typical abnormalities in the strength, rhythm or nature of the pulse: the water-hammer pulse of aortic incompetence or the thready pulse of shock, for example. Again, the examination of the pulse seems to have been elevated into something central to making a diagnosis in every condition.

The nature of traditional Chinese medicine diagnosis

TCM has a remarkable ability to allow apparently contradictory ideas to co-exist. Some authors state that diseases are not 'caused', but are an essential and inevitable component of the individual's pattern (Kaptchuk 1983), while others discuss the causes of disease, just like Western medicine does. Acupuncturists may use terms such as external pathogenic factors, or internal emotional influences such as excessive worry, or behaviour such as an unbalanced diet, or excess of sexual activity as the causes of an illness. Some practitioners will work with the concept of five phases, whereas others will use the modern TCM concept of 'syndromes', i.e. relatively constant pattern of symptoms and a formula for treating them. For example, a stiff and painful neck with rapid onset and changeable symptoms might be due to pathogenic 'Wind' (Maciocia 1989). This is summed up as the idea of 'root and branch' treatment: root treatment is supposed to address the patient's fundamental 'imbalance', but branch treatment only deals with the symptoms.

There follows a list of some of the diagnostic approaches that can be used (Table 8.1), separately or together, to explain the symptoms that any particular patient presents.

These diagnostic methods of TCM need to be tested for reliability, in the sense that different practitioners applying them to particular patients should agree on the diagnosis. We would not be surprised if there is some agreement because, after all, they are systematic methods of classifying medical symptoms and signs. For example, the TCA diagnoses made in women with 'idiopathic' infertility (i.e. cause unknown to Western medicine) showed some reliability in distinguishing them from those with other causes (Coyle & Smith 2005). It does not follow that TCA diagnosis is 'reliable' in the sense of confirming, for example, that Spleen deficiency is a meaningful diagnosis in a case of vaginal discharge.

TABLE 8.1

Examples of traditional diagnostic methods

Diagnostic method	Explanation and/or example
Five phases	Imbalance of one (or more) elements, e.g. dizziness and headaches from insufficient Wood
Organ syndrome	Symptoms due to disturbance of an organ's function, such as lassitude and loose stools from Spleen deficiency
Disturbance in Qi, Blood or Body fluids	What we might refer to as internal medicine, e.g. nausea and vomiting due to 'rebellious Qi'
Eight principles	Diagnosis by Interior/Exterior, Hot/Cold, Full/Empty, and Yin/Yang character of the disease, e.g. pale face, tiredness and lack of appetite from Empty Qi
Meridians and collaterals	Symptoms explained by the pathway of a meridian, e.g. the symptoms of vaginal discharge, cold feeling along the meridian and leg pain indicate a disturbance of the Spleen meridian
Pathogenic factors, from the climate	Aversion to cold, sneezing and runny nose due to an invasion of Wind

We accept that TCM diagnosis may be able to make more subtle differentiations between types of patient than the diagnostic methods of Western medicine. For example, Western doctors may talk about different 'types' of patient, but do not have a terminology or system for codifying them. This is an aspect of TCM that could be well worth exploring in some detail.

Traditional Chinese treatment

Point selection

In classical TCM the acupuncturist selects the points according to their actions, matching these points exactly to the individual patient's diagnosis. Here are three examples from a standard text (Maciocia 1989):

- BL62 (just below the external malleolus) 'benefits the eyes, relaxes sinews, clears the mind and eliminates interior Wind'
- SP10 (just above the knee) 'cools the Blood, regulates menstruation'
- LI11 (lateral border of elbow) 'expels exterior Wind, clears Heat, resolves Dampness and benefits the sinews and joints'.

One can only speculate on how these particular activities ever became attached to individual points: presumably, it was a result of observing the general effects we have discussed in Chapter 5 and some creative interpretation.

The use of this rationale for choosing points for needling seems to us to be a central and significant problem in applying TCM. This is a fundamentally important principle of TCM that is desperately awaiting some kind of supporting evidence.

Needle manipulation

In line with the idea of influencing the flow of *qi* in the meridian, some practitioners use particular needle manipulations, such as clockwise or anticlockwise rotation, and strong as opposed to gentle, supposedly to increase ('reinforce') or decrease ('drain') the *qi*. While the speed of rotation could stimulate nerve endings differentially, it is difficult to imagine that opposite directions of rotation have different effects. After removing the needle, some acupuncturists place their finger over the hole, 'to stop the *qi* escaping'.

Claims of holism

Traditional acupuncturists generally claim that they are practising 'holistically', because their diagnosis can take account of a variety of factors in the patient, such as their food preferences, frequency of sexual intercourse, and the effect of weather on the symptoms. However, holistic medicine is truly a function of the overall approach of the practitioner, not of any system of medicine. There is nothing inherently more holistic in TCA diagnosis than in a comprehensive Western medical assessment: in fact, a good Western medical assessment may well be more holistic in taking greater account of psychological and social factors in a case, which hardly feature in TCA. No system of medicine can claim a monopoly on holism.

Traditional Chinese and Western medical acupuncture

The traditional theories of acupuncture have been challenged in the West by various authors in the UK (Baldry 1993, Campbell 2001, Filshie & White 1998, Mann 1992) and the USA (Ulett 1992). We limit ourselves to some general observations and some rather speculative comments.

Despite a considerable amount of research to try to explain the *meridians* or channels – as nerves, electrical pathways, conduits of sound, pathways in the collagen matrix – there is no evidence to support their existence as physical structures. They are much better explained as a way of understanding common clinical observations such as pain from nerve-root entrapment like sciatica, pressure on other nerves such as the greater occipital nerve, referred sensations from trigger points, or the red lines of ascending lymphangitis, as well as propagated needle sensation that is likely to be due to spinal-cord interconnections. Symptom patterns in one region may have generated the idea that meridians run throughout the body to make a complete and coherent pattern.

There are many concepts in classical acupuncture which can easily be understood as a way of interpreting everyday observations in different terminology. For example, diseases are considered to first invade superficially and then, if unchecked, to invade the internal organs: this could simply reflect observations such as:

- a cold starts in the nose and throat; it may lead to pneumonia in the lungs
- with increasing age, musculoskeletal conditions become more common; serious internal diseases follow later – such as heart attacks, tuberculosis or cancer.

Similarly, back pain is commonly attributed to 'stagnation of *qi* in the Kidneys'. Stagnation of *qi* is probably what we would call muscle spasm, and in patients with back pain, spasm often occurs where the kidneys are situated. This diagnosis of stagnation may be little more than a description of what is observed, and not an indication of kidney disease. These concepts serve to reinforce the convictions of classical TCM acupuncturists, but they cannot be used to provide an argument in favour of classical acupuncture when they can be explained perfectly rationally.

Some more general comments can be added here about the classical (Chinese) interpretation of acupuncture. One problem with acupuncture is that so many different forms of diagnosis are still used, long after the world view on which they are based has been discarded. Different schools of TCA seem to differ in their treatment approaches, but probably all have very similar results in clinical practice. Given what we now know about the widespread effects of stimulating the body with a needle anywhere within quite a large area, it seems that the only rational conclusion is that the actual traditional diagnosis is probably not that important, but that stimulating the patient with a needle is.

Seen from the Western, scientific perspective, acupuncture seems to be a relatively straightforward therapy, given our knowledge of the structure and function of the body. It seems unnecessary to complicate it with elaborate theories. The Western approach to acupuncture is often dismissed as an oversimplification of the original therapy, limited to the treatment of symptoms. Classical acupuncture in contrast claims to 'correct fundamental imbalances' (Table 8.2). We have seen no evidence to convince us that this 'correction of fundamental imbalances' is any more than a combination of generalized beneficial effects on brain centres (as discussed in Chapter 6) together with the patient's expectation of success. Many ancient descriptions of acupuncture actually seem to regard it as treatment of symptoms, not the root cause (Birch & Kaptchuk 1999). Even the *Yellow Emperor's Internal Classic* stated that acupuncture was really only suitable for superficial symptoms, and that internal diseases required herbs. The way we apply acupuncture may actually be more in line with ancient tradition than the TCM approach!

TABLE 8.2

A summary of the principal differences between Western medical acupuncture and traditional Chinese acupuncture

Traditional Chinese medicine	Western medical acupuncture
Theory	
Acts on *qi*	Acts on nerve and muscle
Corrects underlying imbalances	Cannot treat the underlying cause of diseases
'Meridians' are of fundamental importance, and their names are meaningful	Meridian names are only useful labels
High regard for accumulated clinical traditions	High regard for empirical evidence
Integrates new understandings into the old	Self-correcting, rejecting ideas when they become obsolete
Indication	
Effective for any condition	Effective only for certain types of condition
Practice	
Traditional Chinese diagnosis	Conventional Western diagnosis
Points precisely located	Points are general guidelines to appropriate stimulation sites
Individualized therapy, emphasis on point location	Individualized therapy, emphasis mostly on stimulation

Finally, there is the manner in which the understanding of a therapy grows over time. Traditional acupuncture evolved through the unchallenged opinions of experts. It was assumed that these experts had gained accurate knowledge and deep understanding from a lifetime of self-critical observation and experiment. This assumption is probably wrong, since according to our current understanding of 'clinical impressions' compared with 'evidence-based medicine', the so-called 'medical experts' are often wrong.

We prefer to understand as well as we can now, but to be prepared to ditch our ideas when new evidence comes along.

Summary

Acupuncture is usually thought of as originating in China, with the earliest records from about 2000 years ago. However, there are suggestions that a similar practice may have existed in Europe approximately 5000 years ago. The Chinese traditional practice varied over geography and time, and evolved over many centuries during many changes of world views, retaining concepts from each period. In China, acupuncture was gradually rejected in favour of Western medicine from the 17th century, but interest was restored from the 1950s.

Traditionally, Chinese physicians practised with many different models, but after 1950 there was an attempt to unite and modernize the practice, which was called Traditional Chinese Medicine (TCM).

Acupuncture spread to other Eastern nations and subsequently to the West, usually in association with trading links. Acupuncture gained some acceptance among the orthodox medical profession at various periods in history, the most recent beginning in the last half of the 20th century. Traditional concepts include *qi*, *yin* and *yang*, five phases (elements), and meridians. Traditional Chinese understanding of structure and function was impressive in its day, but has not changed in the light of scientific discoveries, and appears outdated and erroneous. Diagnosis in traditional Chinese acupuncture may use several models at the same time, and treatment relies on activating the specific properties that points are supposed to have. A rational approach based on knowledge obtained scientifically can explain many of the concepts of TCM.

Further reading

Kendall D E 2002 Dao of Chinese medicine: understanding an ancient healing art. Oxford, New York

This book claims to show the truth (Dao) about traditional Chinese medicine, by reinterpreting the Chinese explanations in the light of subsequent biomedical discoveries. It is stimulating and knowledgeable, even though some find it ultimately unconvincing, and recommended reading for anyone interested in exploring the field.

Lu G-D, Needham J 2002 Celestial lancets: a history and rationale of acupuncture and moxa. Routledge Curzon, London and New York

This work is part of the major project 'Science and Civilisation' in China of enormous breadth and scholarship to which the authors devoted their lives at the Needham Institute in Cambridge. It is essential and very accessible reading for anyone seriously interested in Chinese medicine. The original publication in 1980 has been republished with an introduction by Vivienne Lo, which discusses research since 1980, including texts discovered since the 1970s, and suggests ways in which the original interpretations may need to be modified. For example, needling the body was originally associated with lancing abscesses; the idea that sharp stones were the forerunner of acupuncture with needles is shown to be far from convincing; and the theoretical foundation of acupuncture and moxibustion could not have occurred before the first century BC. However, as Lo herself comments, the original text is 'unlikely to be superseded'.

Schnorrenberger C 2003 Chen-Chiu, the original acupuncture: a new healing paradigm. Wisdom Publications, Somerville MA

The author is a German physician who has been studying Chinese medicine since the 1970s and has published a number of works in German and English. This book is a summary of his approach to Chinese medicine, in particular the way that he believes the original concepts of Chinese medicine were significantly modified in their transition to Western cultures. While some experts might dispute some of the authors' conclusions, the book remains a useful insight into Chinese medicine.

SECTION 2 THE EVIDENCE BASE

CHAPTER

9

Clinical research into the effectiveness of acupuncture

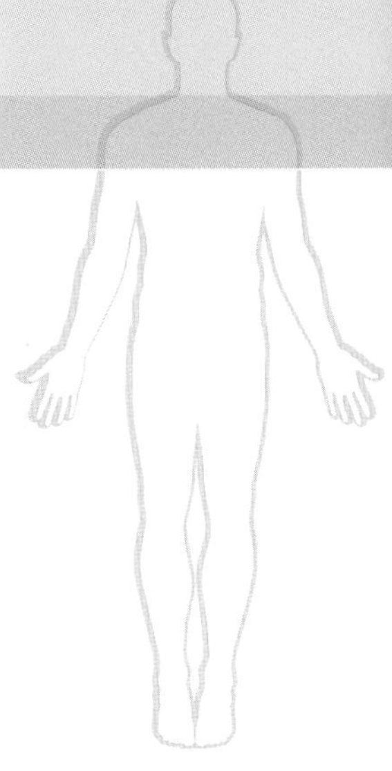

Contents

After reading this chapter you should be able to:

- state three conditions that have good evidence for the effectiveness of acupuncture
- describe three problems in conducting RCTs of acupuncture.

Introduction

Acupuncturists will probably need to provide evidence that acupuncture is effective, safe and cost effective before it can be formally integrated into the policy of any national health service. This does not mean that provision of acupuncture should be forbidden until this evidence is complete and overwhelming – that would risk denying patients a potentially very useful treatment. Individual healthcare practitioners make decisions about using acupuncture or referring patients for treatment on other kinds of evidence: anecdotal reports about the successes of a local practitioner, published case series and audits from local clinics, the views of their colleagues and opinion leaders, and, of course, the wishes of the patient. We are currently in a kind of intermediate situation: there is plenty of evidence that acupuncture is likely to be more valuable than other treatments for patients with a particular problem, but not yet enough evidence to convince policy makers to pay for it.

This chapter will focus on research into effectiveness and will mention the few studies on cost effectiveness that are available; evidence on the safety of acupuncture is discussed in the following chapter.

Rigorous research into acupuncture is not easy. Acupuncture is a complex intervention and when considering ways to investigate it we have to think more of the methods used in research into surgery or physical therapy interventions rather than into drugs, particularly the difficulties of blinding the practitioner and the patients. Here, we shall briefly introduce some of the problems in acupuncture research and the ways of interpreting the results of studies with various control groups, before summarizing the findings of the research in different conditions.

Blinding participants in acupuncture trials

Problems with 'placebo' acupuncture

One of the biggest problems in acupuncture research is that there is really no ideal placebo for acupuncture needles. Placebos are important in research into any therapy for two reasons: (1) to show that the treatment has a *specific* effect (i.e. an effect 'beyond placebo'); only if the treatment is shown to be better than placebo can we argue convincingly that its effect is not just due to the power of expectation or the therapeutic relationship; and (2) to allow blinding or 'masking' of the patients, so that they are not biased when they are asked to assess the effects of treatment. It is acceptable to use a masked observer instead, to remove the bias, but this is not possible for the kind of conditions that acupuncture is mostly used for, since assessment has to rely on the report of the patients themselves.

A placebo must be indistinguishable from the real treatment, but it must be inert. Unfortunately, there is no placebo for an acupuncture needle: anything that feels like a needle inevitably has a physiological effect. For many years, researchers have displayed great invention in trying to find inactive controls, but it is now clear that any stimulus on the skin, even just pressure with the blunt end of a needle, can have profound effects on the limbic system when it is being used in a therapeutic context, i.e. pretending to be a real treatment (Pariente et al 2005). While it is true that a sharp, penetrating needle has a greater effect than blunt pressure on the skin – it affects the insula – the fact remains that the blunt pressure will have treatment effects of its own through widespread activation of the limbic system: a blunt needle is not an inactive placebo.

Pressure on the skin given as 'treatment' has an effect on the limbic system.

This creates a problem, which is that the effect of the blunt needle is almost as large as the effect of the real needle (Fig. 9.1). The difference between the two is often much smaller than the difference between a drug and a placebo drug. Therefore, acupuncture studies that are too small, or not very carefully designed, will fail to reveal this small difference. Studies like this could be interpreted as showing that acupuncture has no real effect, when in fact the acupuncture has an effect, but more patients are required to show the effect. This is known as a type 2 error – the failure to reveal an effect that does actually exist, because of inadequate statistical power, usually because the number of subjects is too small.

'Sham' acupuncture

Since there is no such thing as an inactive 'placebo' control for acupuncture, we should use the term 'sham' instead for any control procedure that is used in a trial to try to make the patient think that they have had treatment. This applies in general to treatments that involve some form of physical intervention, such as surgery, manipulation and acupuncture. Not only is the term more accurate, but also it reminds anyone who is reading the report of the

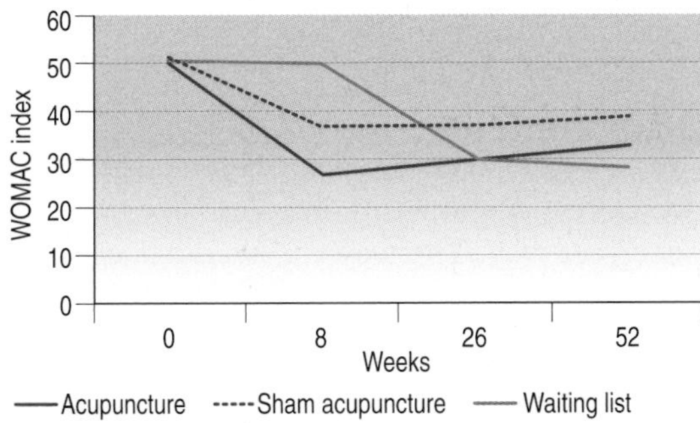

Figure 9.1 Results of a three-armed study showing the response of patients in each arm measured various weeks after the start of the trial; the waiting list group received acupuncture after 8 weeks. The effect of acupuncture is slightly greater than that of placebo, and the difference is statistically significant; both are very much more effective than waiting list. Data taken from an RCT of acupuncture for knee osteoarthritis (Witt C, Brinkhaus B, Jena S et al 2005 acupuncture in patients with osteoarthritis of the knee. Lancet 366: 136–143).

trial that the subjects are receiving an intervention which often has some neurophysiological effect.

A 'placebo-controlled', double-blind trial of acupuncture is technically impossible.

There are two types of sham acupuncture: non-penetrating and penetrating sham.

Non-penetrating sham controls

There is almost no limit to the inventiveness of different researchers in trying to achieve a control that does not penetrate the skin. Some have tried tapping the skin with the guide tube, with a cocktail stick or even with a sharpened fingernail; others have designed a special plastic plug at the end of the guide tube so the needle is driven into the plug and prevented from entering the skin.

Apart from the fact that these devices are active, they are also somewhat limited in the situation in which they can be applied. They can only be used convincingly on points that are out of the patient's line of vision, which effectively means on the back. One way round this problem is to blindfold the patients, or erect some kind of barrier to hide the needling sites.

More recently, researchers have devised a blunted needle, where the shaft is not fixed to the handle so that when you push down on the handle, it simply slides over the shaft rather like a stage dagger. The needle seems to be penetrating the skin, but actually the tip does not penetrate. The needle needs a device to support it if the treatment involves retaining needles for 10 or 20 minutes. In the original version, the Streitberger needle used an adhesive dressing. In the Park device, an extra tube is held in a vertical position by an adhesive flange. Various forms of placebo needle are shown in Plate 8.

These supporting devices themselves cause problems: they may not be easy to use in hairy sites, they need special techniques in practice, and they may interfere with normal needling which also, of course, has to be given using the supporting device, to preserve blinding.

Penetrating sham controls

In many clinical trials, real acupuncture needles have been used in the control group; but in an incorrect way. The way the needle is used 'incorrectly' determines the actual research question. It can be placed:

- in the wrong site – this tests the effect of putting a needle in the correct place; or
- in the right site but only superficially and without stimulation (so called minimal acupuncture) – this tests the effect of deep needle insertion and possibly nerve stimulation; or
- both in the wrong site and superficially – this tests the effects of both site and stimulation.

However, it is difficult to find a 'wrong' site that is credible to the patient, but does not have some effect through segmental analgesia. Patients expect to be needled somewhere near the painful problem, but even superficial needling around the area is likely to have some segmental effect. The difference then between the effects of real and sham treatment could be very small indeed.

Needles in the 'wrong' place can still have segmental and extrasegmental effects.

Finally, it is interesting to note that it may not be very easy for practitioners to give a sham treatment. For example, most acupuncturists have been used to manually stimulating needles ever since they learned acupuncture. It takes quite some concentration to 'unlearn' stimulating the needle in the context of a clinical trial. In a multicentre study in which many practitioners have to unlearn their habits, it is not surprising if the sham treatment is not done very well, and is actually quite strongly active.

Technically, it is easy to apply effective acupuncture, but very difficult to apply an ineffective sham.

Testing the success of patient blinding

Not only should the patients in acupuncture studies be blinded, but that blinding should be verified at the end of the trial, to make sure the control patients have not realized that they have not been given an active treatment. This is a common criticism of acupuncture studies, and yet another difficulty for designing randomized controlled trials (RCTs) with sham acupuncture.

The best way to test blinding is to ask patients directly whether they think they have had real or sham acupuncture. However, this may interfere with the effectiveness of the very treatment that is being tested, by focusing patients' attention on the treatment and reminding them that they might be having a sham treatment. It may even lead them to doubt the treatment they are having, even if it is active.

It is difficult to know when best to pose the question: after the first treatment or two, patients might not have enough experience of the treatment to form an opinion. But at the end of treatment their answer will be influenced by whether they have responded to treatment or not – so in a study where acupuncture is effective, patients will conclude that they have active treatment and the trial will be criticized for failing to ensure blinding!

Verifying patient blinding without interfering with treatment is difficult.

Another solution has been attempted quite often in acupuncture RCTs. Patients are asked to assess how credible the treatments have been, using some indirect questions such as: 'Would you recommend this treatment to a friend?', or 'Would you expect this treatment to work for another condition you had?'. In this way the credibility of the real and the sham treatments can be compared. However, there is a technical weakness in the statistical analysis (it requires test of equivalence not difference), which limits the reliability of this method.

Practitioner blinding

Ideally, in an RCT the acupuncture practitioner should be blinded (masked) to whether the treatment is real or sham. This is difficult, though not impossible. We know of two ways in which researchers have tried to achieve this. In one, the practitioner who performed the treatment was a non-acupuncturist who was trained specially to give two treatments without being told which was active and which was sham (Lagrue et al 1977). The problem with this method is that the practitioner's skill in acupuncture is likely to be inadequate, so that the treatment is not of high quality. In the other method, one acupuncturist examined the patients and devised two treatments for each patient, only one of which was correct (Allen et al 1998). The patients were then randomized to receive one or other treatment from the second practitioner, who theoretically remained blinded to which was the correct one – but in practice might recognize patient types and identify patterns of prescriptions. This method is also very heavy on resources.

For now, we shall have to accept that acupuncturists, like surgeons, cannot readily be blinded in clinical trials. However, participants should be blinded whenever possible and, additionally, the assessors (and those who perform data entry and analysis, ideally) should also be blinded.

Other problems in acupuncture research

Conditions suitable for clinical trials

Several surveys have shown that acupuncture is most commonly used to treat musculoskeletal conditions. It seems particularly effective for these conditions within about 6–12 weeks from the onset, i.e. before they become chronic. However, it is very difficult for researchers to recruit the patients at this intermediate stage. They are probably still being supervised in primary care and primary-care practitioners see a large number of patients with a wide range of conditions: so patients with any particular condition are few and far between. By the time the patients are referred to secondary care, their condition is likely to have become chronic. So there are more patients available for recruitment to the study in secondary care, but their condition will have developed and may well be less responsive to acupuncture treatment.

Conditions that respond best to acupuncture are likely to be difficult to research.

Many trials of acupuncture have been undertaken in secondary care because that is where the resources are – support staff, facilities and patients. But these patients will have already received other treatments for their condition and so they will present a tough test for any treatment. It would be wrong to expect a high success rate. The results of such trials should not be used as the basis for global statements like 'acupuncture does not work'.

Acupuncture research could most profitably concentrate on musculoskeletal injuries, particularly at the stage immediately beyond the time when they might have been expected to heal. Other promising conditions include headache, nausea and vomiting, and osteoarthritis of moderate severity.

It is important to be well informed about the condition that is to be researched, as this may profoundly affect the sort of response that is expected, and so the design of the study. For example, it is becoming clear that affective pain, i.e. the emotional response to pain, responds reasonably well to the limbic system modulation that seems to be a general effect of all forms of acupuncture, including sham acupuncture. Therefore, real acupuncture is likely to be only slightly better than sham acupuncture in conditions such as tension headache and migraine with a large affective component. In contrast, sensory pain may respond better to real acupuncture because it has neuromodulatory effects additional to those on the insula (Lund & Lundeberg 2006). Therefore, one might more confidently design a study to test for a difference between real and sham acupuncture treatment of osteoarthritis of the knee, with its greater sensory component.

Lack of research resources: suboptimal acupuncture treatment

Pharmacological research into new drugs follows a well-trodden research pathway. It starts with careful phase I and II studies to identify the best candidates for the treatment and the best mode of delivery, and only then moves on to rigorous, well-resourced, definitive, clinical trials.

In contrast, most acupuncture trials have been undertaken as one-off studies by enthusiasts who are motivated by the desire to demonstrate to the world that this novel treatment is effective. Often the acupuncture treatments are not standard, and have not been adequately justified, for example by checking the literature or by forming a consensus of expert opinion. For acupuncture studies to have convincing results, we need to know much more about the best details of acupuncture for different conditions. We need to undertake preliminary studies comparing different types of acupuncture to find the best for different types of patient – the equivalent of phase I studies in pharmaceutical research.

Lack of knowledge about the optimal acupuncture for different conditions seriously compromises clinical trials.

Often other aspects of acupuncture studies seem to have set them up to fail. Sample sizes have been inadequate, leading to type 2 errors. Outcome measures have not chosen carefully enough, so they are not appropriate and sensitive enough to show subtle effects; and the statistical analysis may not be the most appropriate for the data, perhaps because it cannot deal with baseline differences between the groups.

Acupuncture as a complex intervention

It will be obvious to the reader who has studied the chapters on acupuncture mechanisms in this book that needles are capable of producing a wide variety of effects. These effects are likely to be different at different times because they depend to a considerable extent on the neurological status of the patient at the time of treatment. For example, the best effects may be seen in patients who are not anxious, and there may be other ways in which the nervous system responds better when it is 'primed'. This becomes all the more complicated because acupuncture can itself alter the status of the patient – by reducing the anxiety, for example.

All these variables, over which we have little control, can affect the response to acupuncture, and there are probably others that we have yet to discover. So, it is no surprise that the responses to acupuncture can vary enormously between two clinical trials even when they appear, to all intents and purposes, identical.

Results of acupuncture trials at odds with clinical observation

The many design problems that we have discussed throughout this chapter all combine to greatly diminish the chance of finding a positive effect of acupuncture. Given this whole range of difficulties that are particular to acupuncture research, and given the lack of research resources in this subject, there are many explanations as to why the results of controlled trials of acupuncture often do not truly reflect the effects that we see every day in practice.

Acupuncturists are convinced of the effectiveness of acupuncture by watching the responses of patients in daily practice – patient reactions that are both completely new to medicine and at the same time repeatedly observed in different patients, such as *de qi* sensation, the rapid relief of pain in certain problems such as myofascial trigger points, the pain relief experienced on the following day in other cases of pain, and the side effects such as drowsiness and euphoria. Acupuncturists are convinced of the value of their therapy despite the rather poor evidence, and feel reassured that better designed studies will produce results that bear out their clinical observations.

Acupuncture is highly effective in clinical practice, but its specific effect is difficult to prove.

In fact, there have recently been some encouraging signs that the quality of acupuncture research is improving, and it is reassuring that many of the newer, more rigorous, better designed studies are producing more convincingly positive results, in conditions as varied as nausea from chemotherapy, neck pain and chronic knee pain. This in turn is reflected in more positive outcomes of the newer systematic reviews, compared with the older reviews, which were often limited by the poor quality of the studies.

Choice of the control group

Acupuncture researchers need to choose the appropriate control group to answer the question they are interested in. We need to remember what that question was when we interpret the results of the controlled trial. The control groups most commonly used are:

- *no additional treatment, e.g. patients on a waiting list*: the question here is whether acupuncture is better than the treatment that patients are already using, such as non-steroidal anti-inflammatory drugs. Almost every time, acupuncture has shown itself superior to usual care for many conditions, often by a considerable margin. Part of this effect will of course be due to the high expectations of acupuncture that patients may have, but that reflects the real situation in clinical practice. So the results are useful in indicating the sort of effects we might see with acupuncture in practice
- *another treatment*: the question here is whether acupuncture is better than other available treatment options, such as spinal manipulation for low back pain. The answer is important for patients and their doctors, in making decisions about planning health care.

These two types of study do not find out whether it is the needles themselves that are effective, or whether it is some other part of the treatment – the patients' expectation, the clinical setting or the physical contact, for example. Sceptics may, therefore, dismiss positive results as 'only a placebo effect', but that is speculative, and shows a lack of understanding of the relevance of research findings. In giving any treatment, the overall effect includes both the specific effect and the expectation, therapeutic relationship and so on. To wait for compelling evidence of an effect 'beyond placebo' before deciding to use a treatment that is known to be safe carries a serious risk of denying patients effective relief of symptoms. It may also cost patients money, for example if they are denied an early return to work.

- *sham acupuncture*: this control group is used in a study designed to find out if acupuncture is superior to *placebo*. This is the kind of study that policy makers want, because they need to know that a treatment 'has a biological effect' before they will consider providing it. Given the practical difficulties of 'placebo acupuncture' that we have discussed in detail already, it is likely that sham-controlled studies with negative results could be unreliable. False-negative results are highly likely. The fact that acupuncture is shown to be much better than usual care or other treatments is much more important for patients than whether it has yet been formally proved superior to 'placebo' in their particular condition. After all, placebo is not a treatment option, whereas usual care or other treatments are what they are going to be offered

- *other placebos*: a few studies have used other placebos as a control – placebo tablets, placebo TENS and so on. These studies are not as helpful as they might appear: if acupuncture is superior to placebo TENS, sceptics could argue that it is because the needles have greater psychological impact. Also, as before, in practice patients are not going to be offered these other placebos, so the results of these studies do not influence practice directly.

The German insurance company studies

In the years following the turn of the 21st century, several German health insurance companies sponsored a series of rigorous studies. These companies had been reimbursing patients for acupuncture treatment, but finding it increasingly expensive. So they decided to seek evidence on which to base their reimbursement decisions, and organized a range of studies using different designs to answer different questions. They ran the studies in patients with headache (tension headache or migraine), neck pain, back pain, and knee and hip osteoarthritis.

They ran large, uncontrolled, observational studies to measure the overall safety and effectiveness of acupuncture, and large RCTs comparing acupuncture with usual care to measure the relative improvements in patients associated with treatment. These showed large treatment effects, and a high level of safety.

They organized three-arm RCTs, giving the groups acupuncture, sham acupuncture with superficial needling to non-traditional points, and leaving one group on a waiting list for subsequent acupuncture treatment (Linde et al 2006, Witt et al 2006a). At the end of treatment, patients who had acupuncture were more improved than those who had sham, in nearly all studies, though in most cases the difference was a trend and only reached statistical significance in the case of osteoarthritis. Both acupuncture and sham acupuncture were significantly better than usual care, for almost every condition tested.

A second programme of larger, three-arm, sham-controlled RCTs (GERAC) used the best standard treatment in the third arm rather than waiting list (e.g. Scharf et al 2006). These trials gave useful data on the value of acupuncture relative to the best standard care at the time.

There has always been some question whether acupuncture used in the context of a clinical trial is more effective than 'everyday' acupuncture in normal clinical practice. The insurance companies took the opportunity of settling that question by conducting a *preference* study (Witt et al 2006b). Patients were invited to join a trial in which they would be randomized to have acupuncture either straight away or after a 3-month wait. Patients who declined to be randomized were offered acupuncture straight away, and they were generally those with slightly more severe symptoms. The most important finding of this study was that the acupuncture was equally effective whether it was given in ordinary practice, outside the RCT, or whether in the context of the RCT. The fact that the response to acupuncture was so stable and predictable (among a group of patients) could be interpreted as another sign that it has a biological effect and is more than 'placebo'.

Reimbursement for acupuncture treatment of chronic knee pain and low back pain is based on evidence.

To summarize these results:

- acupuncture is either equivalent to (migraine), or much better than (chronic low back pain, knee osteoarthritis), standard care
- the effectiveness of acupuncture in RCTs is the same as in everyday practice
- acupuncture generally shows at least a trend to being superior to sham acupuncture, but only reaches statistical significance for knee pain. Bear in mind that sham acupuncture in these studies was very likely to be an active treatment.

On the strength of these results, the insurance organizations decided to provide funding for acupuncture treatment of two conditions:

1. Osteoarthritis of the knee – because it is better than sham acupuncture, and the effect is of a useful size
2. Back pain – because, although acupuncture was not proven to be better than sham acupuncture, low back pain is an economic disaster for which the standard care has little to offer, that it is sufficient that acupuncture proved to be better than standard care.

Assessing the evidence

We shall now summarize the evidence on acupuncture for a range of conditions, using systematic reviews where available and otherwise RCTs.

Given the particular problems in conducting clinical trials of acupuncture, it is hardly surprising that reviewing them also leads to difficulties, and is often not done well. Poor reviews, for example, have combined different conditions in a single review, have failed to define the type of acupuncture or take account of whether it has been performed well, and have failed to understand the subtlety of different sham controls. This inevitably leads to inaccurate results, which are often to the detriment of acupuncture.

We are not presenting an all-inclusive review of the evidence here; for example, we do not consider the laboratory studies in humans, of which there are many. This chapter is intended as an introduction to the strengths and weaknesses of the evidence base of acupuncture. We believe that the evidence here can be thought of as a pointer to the main areas where acupuncture is most likely to be fully integrated into Western medical care.

We shall largely confine this discussion of effectiveness to controlled clinical trials published in the Western literature, since the Chinese literature seems to only contain positive studies (Vickers et al 1998).

We shall consider the evidence about the cost effectiveness of acupuncture in a separate section towards the end of this chapter.

Acupuncture for musculoskeletal conditions

Neck pain

Neck pain is a condition which, according to many practitioners' clinical experience, seems to respond more quickly and satisfactorily than almost any other. The current Cochrane review of 10 trials of acupuncture (661 participants) for chronic neck pain concludes:

> *There is moderate evidence that acupuncture relieves pain better than some sham treatments, measured at the end of the treatment. There is moderate evidence that those who received acupuncture reported less pain at short-term follow-up than those on a waiting list. There is also moderate evidence that acupuncture is more effective than inactive treatments for relieving pain post treatment and this is maintained at short-term follow-up.*
>
> *(Trinh et al 2007)*

Considering that a Cochrane review has to couch its conclusions in extremely cautious and highly circumspect language, and considering also the difficulties in acupuncture research, this statement actually amounts to quite a significant endorsement of acupuncture. When we look at this evidence in the context of other reviews (below, chronic low back pain) showing that acupuncture is superior to sham treatment for spinal pain elsewhere, it seems reasonable to conclude that acupuncture has specific effects on neck pain.

The size of the effect of acupuncture in chronic neck pain is not particularly large, but since other treatments also have limited effect, there is certainly a place for acupuncture in managing this condition. Furthermore, the large German Acupuncture in Routine Care (ARC) study on neck pain (N = 14 161 total cohort; N = 3766 randomized), which more accurately reflects what happens in actual practice, clearly demonstrates the effectiveness of acupuncture compared with usual care (Witt et al 2006a). Note the size of the randomized element of this trial compared with the total number of participants in the Cochrane review mentioned above (Trinh et al 2007).

In primary care, patients usually present with acute or subacute neck pain. There are no RCTs specifically on this group, but evidence from primary care shows that patients respond quickly and satisfactorily (Ross et al 1999).

Upper limb pain

One good-quality study in patients in a sports centre with rotator cuff tendonitis ($N = 52$) was conducted by Streitberger and colleagues, who first described the collapsing, non-penetrating sham needle (Kleinhenz et al 1999). The status of the shoulder condition was assessed by blinded orthopaedic surgeons using a standardized assessment (Constant-Murley score) for pain and function. After 4 weeks' treatment with acupuncture, the improvement was 19 points, but after sham acupuncture it was only 8 points ($P = 0.014$).

Tennis elbow (lateral epicondylitis) often responds in clinical practice so could be a good candidate for research, and it is surprising that there are so few studies on this subject. Two studies were positive. In the first ($N = 82$), Haker and colleagues found deep needling at acupuncture points was more effective than superficial needling at the same points (Haker & Lundeberg 1990). In a second study ($N = 55$), Fink and colleagues found ten treatments (twice per week) with genuine acupuncture were superior to needling at inappropriate sites, when the patients were assessed 2 weeks after the end of treatment (Fink et al 2002). In both studies, the difference did not remain statistically significant at the long-term follow-up, which probably reflects the fact that tennis elbow resolves over time anyway. Trinh and colleagues reviewed six high-quality studies and concluded that they amounted to strong evidence that acupuncture had at least a short-term effect on lateral epicondylitis (Trinh et al 2004).

Low back pain

A systematic review found 33 studies of acupuncture for low back pain – a quantity of research which one might expect to produce definitive conclusions (Manheimer et al 2005). However, the studies recruited patients with various of types of back pain, various types of acupuncture, and a range of outcomes, so each individual analysis included a relatively small number of studies and tended to have somewhat inconclusive findings.

Acupuncture was significantly superior to sham treatment (seven trials) and to usual care (eight trials) for the short-term effect on chronic back pain. The effect sizes were reasonable – 0.5 and 0.7 respectively. There are not enough studies to be sure about improvement in function, or about the long-term results in pain, though in both cases the trends were strongly in favour of acupuncture. Similar conclusions were drawn by a Cochrane Review published at about the same time (Furlan et al 2005).

Since those reviews, a study has been published from primary care in the UK ($N = 239$), which compared acupuncture with usual care alone. Acupuncture was superior for one of the measurements of pain, showing a trend at 12 months and a significant difference at 24 months (Thomas et al 2005). However, there was no difference between the groups in the assessment of impairment of function, using the Oswestry score.

Overall, then, acupuncture has a role to play in managing chronic back pain. Its success rate may not be too impressive, but is quite respectable in comparison with other treatments. The German insurance companies decided to reimburse acupuncture for back pain for that very reason.

Low back and pelvic pain in pregnancy

Some authorities insist on differentiating spinal back pain from pelvic pain in pregnant women. Not all the studies have done this, so it is not easy to combine them meaningfully in a review. In fact, the majority of studies have shown a good result whatever the origin of the pain, though the studies have been unblinded. For example, in one study in 60 women, acupuncture was superior to physiotherapy in relieving pain and disability (Wedenberg et al 2000). Another study was based in Gothenburg and involved 386 pregnant women with pelvic girdle pain, who all received standard treatment (Elden et al 2005). Women who received acupuncture in addition had significantly reduced pain, and acupuncture was also superior to specific stabilizing exercises.

Chronic knee pain

A recent systematic review found 13 RCTs (involving 2362 patients) of acupuncture for chronic knee pain, mainly due to osteoarthritis (White et al 2007). The authors set the following five criteria for whether the acupuncture was deemed to be 'adequate':

- At least six treatments
- At least once per week
- At least four points needled
- For at least 20 minutes
- Either manual stimulation to elicit *de qi* or electrical stimulation of sufficient intensity to produce more than minimal sensation.

In addition, they specified that sham controls could only be called 'true sham' if they avoided needling in the legs in the same segments as the knee joint. A meta-analysis showed that acupuncture was clearly superior to sham acupuncture for both pain and function, both in the short term and over a period of 6–12 months.

The results are robust: they rely on good-quality studies performed in different research centres, in different countries and are not influenced by differences between the studies (the technical word for which is heterogeneity). To evaluate the actual clinical value of the acupuncture treatment, these authors calculated the 'effect size' of treatment. The effect size is the difference that is observed, divided by the standard deviation, and this simple calculation gives a number (without any units) that can be used to compare treatments. Usually, effect sizes of 0.2 are regarded as small, 0.5 are medium and 0.8 are large. The effect size of acupuncture compared with usual care is estimated at 0.8. The effect size compared with placebo is about 0.3, which is approximately the same as the effect of non-steroidal anti-inflammatory drugs (White & Kawakita 2006).

This review includes four modern, well-designed studies, which were in total agreement in showing acupuncture to be superior to conservative treatment for knee pain, such as usual care or education. Three of the studies also found acupuncture superior to sham acupuncture, whereas the largest study (Scharf et al 2006) did not. This one found only a trend in favour of acupuncture in the percentage of responders to real and to sham acupuncture, which did not reach statistical difference. The reasons for this study only showing a trend could include: (1) in this large multicentre study involving nearly 300 practitioners, each practitioner treated an average of only three patients, so was unlikely to have given optimum treatment, whether real or sham acupuncture; (2) all groups were given exercise, which may operate in a similar way to acupuncture, reducing the combined effect; and (3) measuring the percentage of responders is less sensitive than measuring changes in pain scores. In reality, the results of this study were directly in line with the other studies in the meta-analysis (Fig. 9.2), which concluded that:

- acupuncture is superior to sham acupuncture for chronic knee pain
- acupuncture's benefits for pain and function last more than 6 months
- in view of acupuncture's advantages, such as safety and no need for a daily dose, it should be considered as a genuine alternative to NSAIDs.

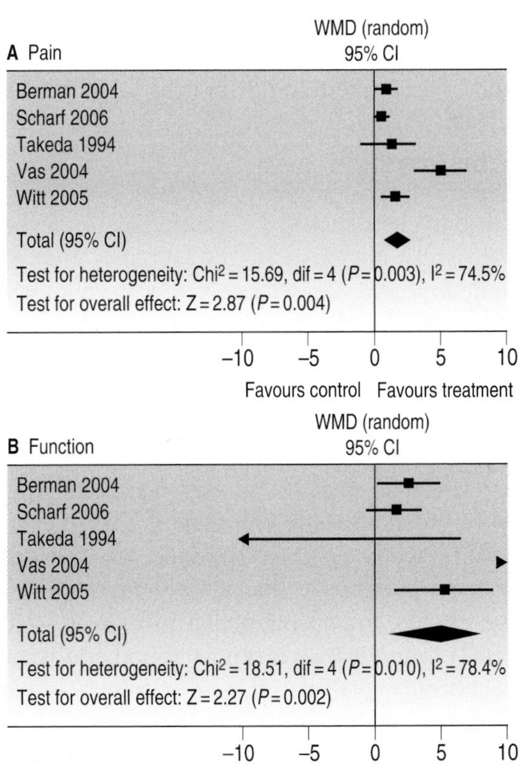

Figure 9.2 Meta-analysis of acupuncture compared with sham acupuncture for chronic knee pain. (White A, Foster N, Cummings M, Barlas P 2006 The effectiveness of acupuncture for osteoarthritis of the Knee – a systematic review. Acupuncture in Medicine 24(Suppl): S40–S48. Reproduced from Acupuncture in Medicine 2007, with permission.)

Myofascial pain

In clinical practice, certain types of myofascial pain, after injury for example, respond most rapidly to acupuncture and are one of the most satisfying conditions to treat. We might, therefore, expect to find plenty of research into it. There are a number of studies, but they are rather difficult to interpret because often it is not clear how carefully the patients have been diagnosed. Rather few of the studies seem to have treated patients with straightforward post-traumatic myofascial pain, and most have included patients with myofascial trigger points that are secondary to other degenerative conditions. This confusion over the diagnosis has been demonstrated in a review (Tough et al 2007). Tenderness is common in patients with pain, but tenderness does not necessarily equate with a true MTrP.

Edwards and Knowles examined patients who were referred by their GP for physiotherapy, and selected those ($N = 40$) with trigger points, diagnosed by spot tenderness, pain recognition and limitation of movement. One group had superficial needling and was taught stretching exercises; another group had stretching exercises alone; and a third group had no treatment (Edwards & Knowles 2003). There was a trend in favour of acupuncture at all follow-up periods, but the difference was only significantly superior ($P = 0.043$) to stretch alone at 3 weeks after treatment. They also measured the pressure pain threshold over the trigger points, and found similar changes. A larger study might well show a significant difference (false-negative result, type 2 error).

Ceccherelli and colleagues found a positive effect in favour of deep needling when compared with superficial needling in patients with shoulder pain ($N = 44$): there was a significant difference in favour of deep needling at the end of treatment and 3 months later (Ceccherelli et al 2001).

Fibromyalgia

Fibromyalgia should be clearly distinguished from myofascial trigger point pain, most obviously by the fact that myofascial trigger point pain is generally unilateral and has relatively few psychological consequences. Fibromyalgia is diagnosed by the presence of pain above and below the waist and on both sides of the body for at least 3 months, with tenderness to pressure at 11 of 18 defined points. Ninety-six per cent of patients with fibromyalgia also have fatigue, and 86% insomnia (Wolfe et al 1990).

The literature on acupuncture for fibromyalgia was reviewed some years ago (Berman et al 1999). Seven studies (three RCTs and four cohort studies) were included: only one was of high methodological quality. This one high-quality study ($N = 70$) found that real electroacupuncture over 3 weeks was more effective than sham acupuncture for relieving pain, increasing pain thresholds, improving global ratings and reducing morning stiffness (Deluze 1992). Some patients reported no benefit, and some reported an exacerbation of fibromyalgia-related pain – which is commonly observed when treating such patients in clinical practice.

A more recent, sham-controlled RCT was also unusually rigorous, and included features such as placing a board under the patient's chin to prevent them seeing the treatment (Martin et al 2006). In two groups of 25 patients, electroacupuncture was significantly better than sham acupuncture according to the Fibromyalgia Impact Questionnaire over the 7-month trial period. Fatigue and anxiety greatly improved.

Therefore, acupuncture may be helpful for some patients with fibromyalgia, though the evidence is not conclusive.

Other musculoskeletal conditions

There are few trials on acupuncture for osteoarthritis (OA) of the hip, but the large pragmatic study from the German insurance company series found that the effects of acupuncture on hip pain were similar to the effects on knee pain (Witt et al 2006b). There is not enough evidence from RCTs to draw any useful conclusions about the role of acupuncture in treating inflammatory arthritis, such as ankylosing spondylitis or rheumatoid arthritis.

Acupuncture for headache

Migraine

The majority of studies in migraine have investigated the role of acupuncture in prevention, i.e. treatment given in between attacks. A review of sixteen RCTs of acupuncture for prevention of migraine concluded that the balance of evidence is in favour of acupuncture being superior to sham, although the overall quality of the studies was too weak to draw strong conclusions (Melchart et al 2001).

Since that review was conducted, one large RCT has been published in which patients with chronic headache ($N = 401$, mainly with migraine) were randomized either to receive 12 acupuncture treatments or simply to continue usual GP care (Vickers et al 2004). Over the 1 year's follow-up the acupuncture group experienced 22 fewer days with headache than the control group. The difference was significant. The acupuncture group also reported lower headache scores and better quality of life. The improvement was associated with a reduction in use of healthcare resources which offset some of the cost of the acupuncture treatment (see below). This trial was funded as part of the UK health service's Health Technology Assessment programme.

The German insurance series included two large RCTs that have been published. In one, 12 treatments of acupuncture were compared with sham acupuncture (superficial needling of non points) and waiting list, in 302 patients with migraine (Linde et al 2005). Both interventions were significantly ($P = 0.001$) better than waiting list control for days with moderate or severe headache, but there was no significant difference between real and sham acupuncture. In the other trial, acupuncture was compared with sham acupuncture and with standard medication with β-blockers, calcium-channel blockers or antiepileptic drugs in 960 patients (Diener et al 2006). There was no significant difference in the days with migraine in the groups after treatment, though a trend in favour of acupuncture with response rates of 47% in the real acupuncture group, 39% in the sham acupuncture group and 40% in the standard group.

The question whether acupuncture has any value in the treatment of *acute* migraine was studied in one trial ($N = 179$), which compared acupuncture with injection of sumatriptan and with a sham injection (Melchart et al 2003). If given in the early stages, acupuncture and sumatriptan both blocked the development of full-blown migraine in 35% of patients, whereas sham did so in only 18%. However, if the first treatment failed and the headache became established, then sumatriptan was more effective than acupuncture. Acupuncture caused significantly fewer side effects than sumatriptan.

Tension-type headache

Chronic tension headache – defined as headache that occurs more than 15 days a month – is an almost intractable condition and a hard test for acupuncture. Headaches that occur on less than 15 days a month (classified as episodic tension headaches) do respond to some interventions, including acupuncture. In some patients tension headache symptoms may be closely linked to TrPs in the shoulders and neck, and it may be these patients who respond best to treatment. A systematic review of acupuncture in tension headache reached a 'promising' verdict since one study was positive and another showed a positive trend (Melchart et al 2001).

Since that review's publication, other studies have not been supportive. One study ($N = 50$) found no difference between needling tender points and pressure with a cocktail stick (White et al 2000), again possibly explained by limbic system effects. In another study, 69 patients received either traditional acupuncture or sham needling, with no significant difference in outcome (Karst et al 2001) – but patients with chronic tension headache were included in this study.

Another study, this one within the German insurance series, included 270 patients with episodic or chronic tension-type headache (Melchart et al 2005). They received either acupuncture or superficial needling at non-acupuncture points, or were within a waiting list control group. Again, both forms of acupuncture were significantly better than waiting list for reducing the number of days with headache. There was a strong trend in favour of acupuncture, shown by the responder rate: the proportion of responders (at least 50% reduction in days with headache) was 46% in the acupuncture group, 35% in the minimal acupuncture group, and 4% in the waiting list group.

It seems likely that studies that select patients more carefully – i.e. only moderate severity and with symptoms clearly related to trigger points – may have more chance of positive results.

Acupuncture for other painful conditions

Chronic pain

An exhaustive systematic review of the literature found a total of 51 studies published in English in which acupuncture was used for chronic pain, including musculoskeletal conditions, Raynaud's syndrome, angina, post-herpetic neuralgia,

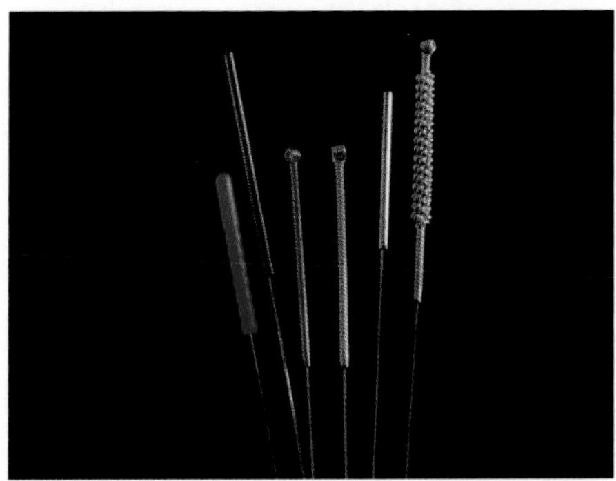

Plate 1 Acupuncture needles showing the development of different types of handle over several years. The old-fashioned double-wound solid silver was superseded by wound silver, then stainless steel or copper and more recently plastic.

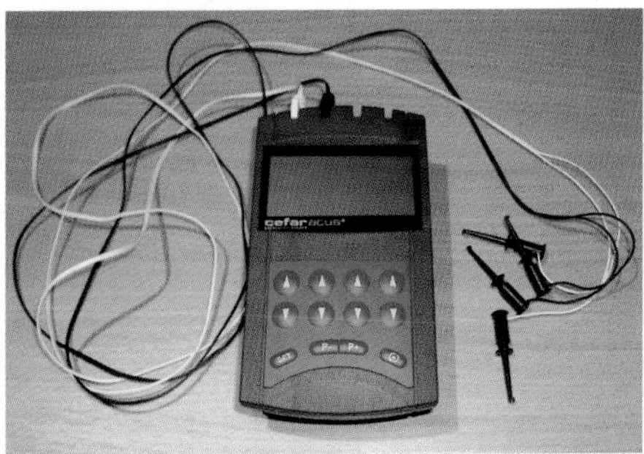

Plate 2 An example of a typical modern electroacupuncture stimulator, which is used to stimulate needles in Western acupuncture instead of the strong manual stimulation that was used by Chinese acupuncturists.

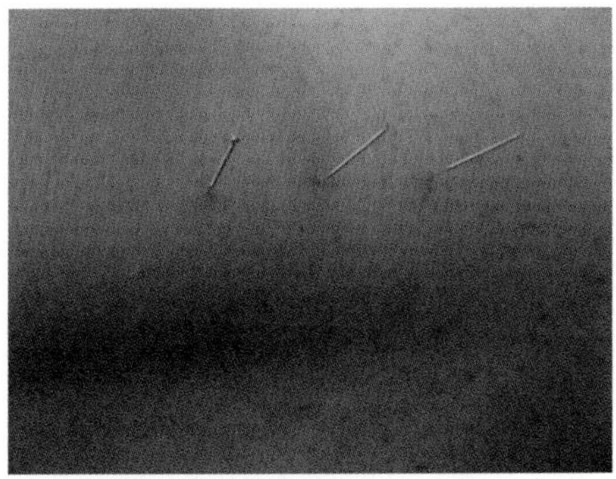

Plate 3 Flares developing in the tissues surrounding a needle, which indicate that the local blood supply is increased through a local nerve reflex.

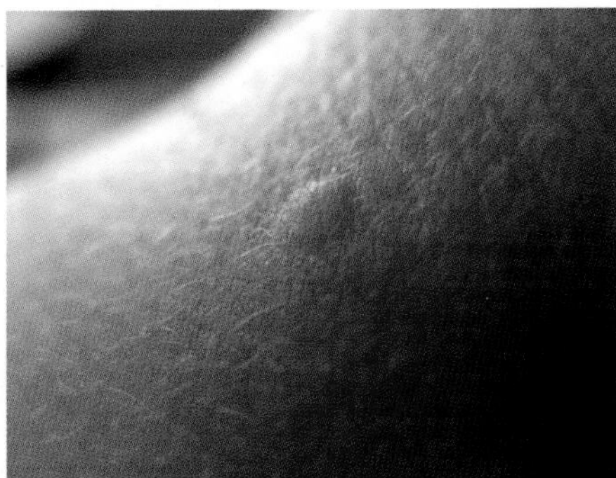

Plate 4 Close-up view of a weal after removal of the acupuncture needle. The weal is the result of fluid leakage from the small blood vessels – another sign of the local response to acupuncture.

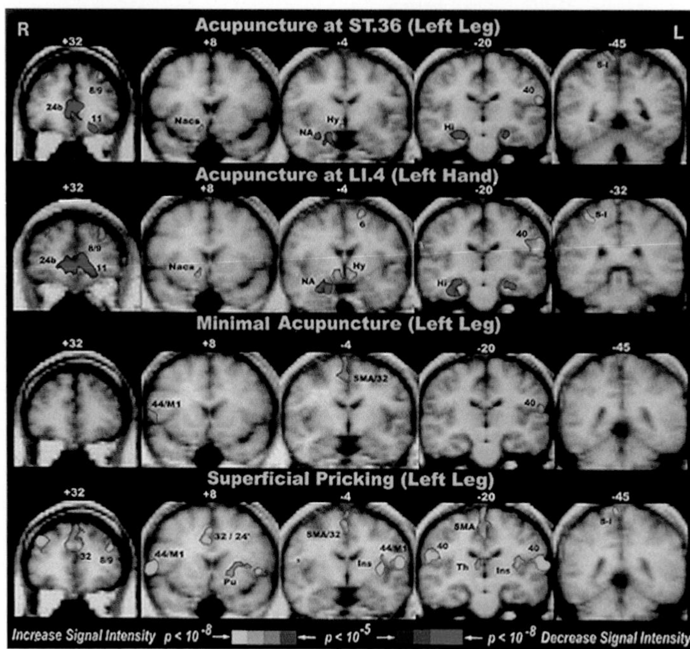

Plate 5 Functional magnetic resonance image of brain activation showing response of various limbic system centres in nine patients given acupuncture at LI4, acupuncture at ST36, minimal acupuncture (superficial needling over an acupuncture point) or superficial pricking elsewhere. Yellow-red colours indicate increased activity of nucleus accumbens (Nacs) and hypothalamus (Hy) as well as areas in sensory cortex. Green-blue colours indicate decreased activity at amygdala (NA) and hippocampus (Hi). Numbers above each image indicate distance in mm from anterior commissure. Numbers in cortical areas of the images correspond to Brodmann areas. (Reproduced from Wu et al Radiology 1999; 212(1): 133–141 with permission of the publishers)

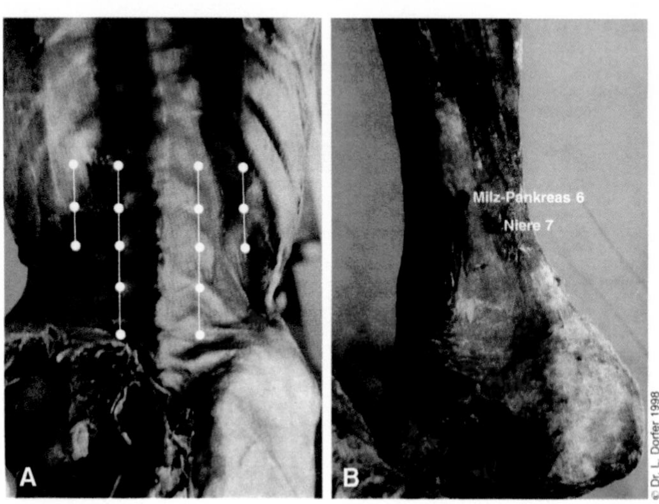

Plates 6 A and B Photographs of the body of Ötzi (the Ice Man) showing (A) tattoos on the back in strikingly similar location to the classical acupuncture points that have been superimposed; and (B) tattoos on the medial aspect of the lower leg in the location of SP6 (Milz-Pankreas 6) and KI7 (Niere 7). (Reproduced with kind permission of Dr L Dorfer)

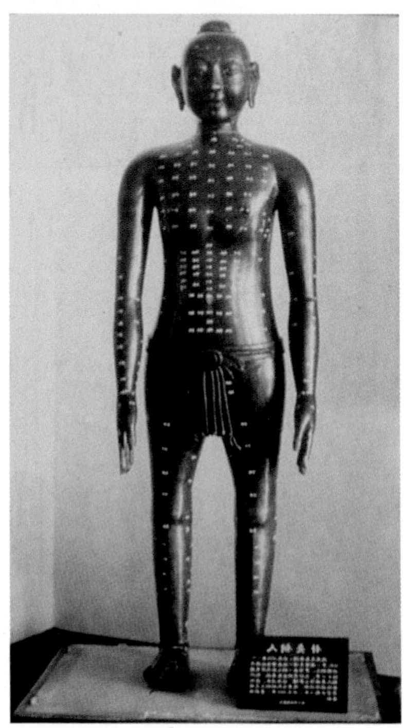

Plate 7 Hollow bronze statue showing acupuncture points. This is a photograph of a reproduction of the original statue, cast in 1443 AD during the Ming Dynasty.

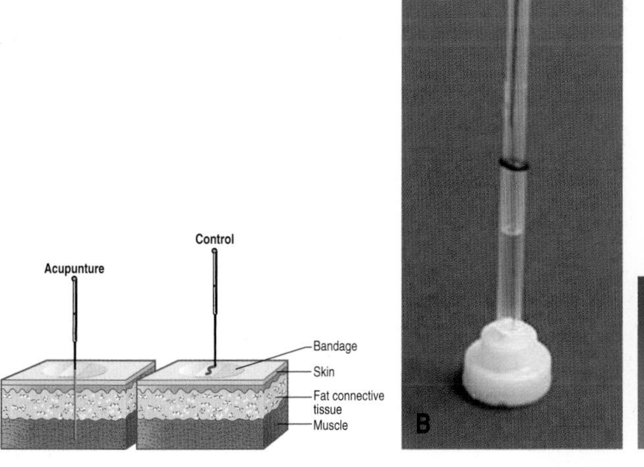

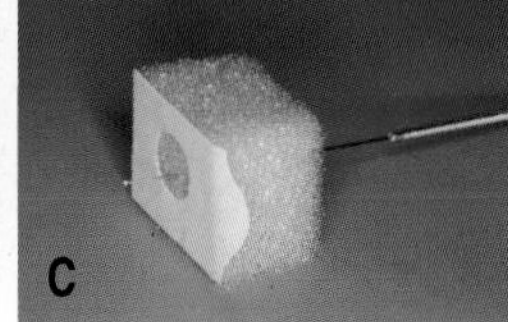

Plates 8 A, B and C Various forms of placebo device and support: (A) Streitberger needle supported by adhesive dressing (reproduced with permission from Martin et al Mayo Clin Proc 2006; 81(6): 749–757); (B) Park needle supported by guide tube and adhesive flange (reproduced with kind permission of Dr Jongbae Park); (C) Blunt needle with adhesive surgical foam as support (reproduced with kind permission of Dr Mathias Fink).

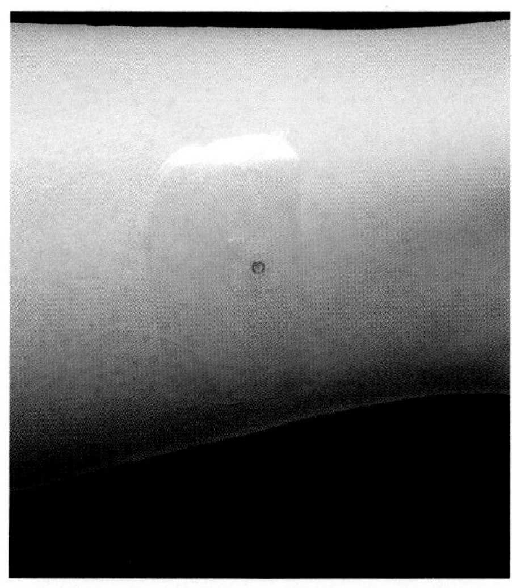

Plate 9 Photograph of indwelling needles with 2 mm projection.

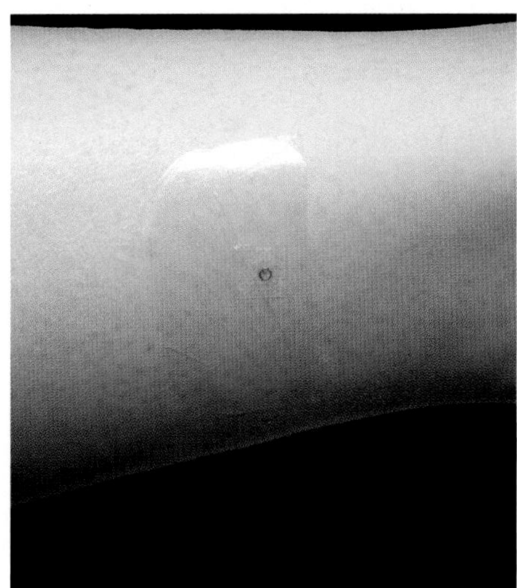

Plate 10 Indwelling acupuncture needle supplied with adhesive plaster.

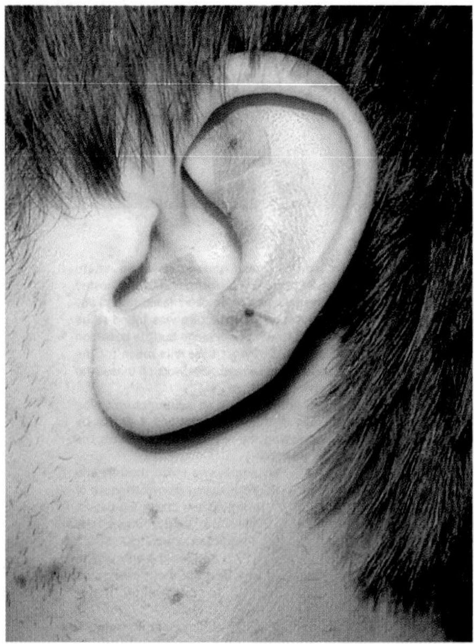

Plate 11 Photograph of *Vaccaria* seeds used for auricular stimulation.

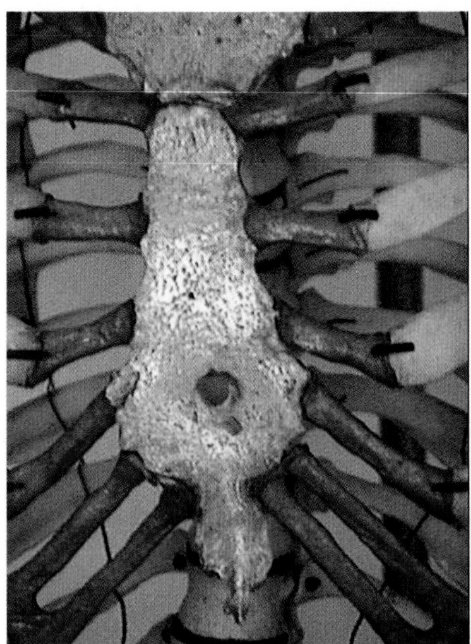

Plate 12 Photograph of foramen sternale. (With kind permission of Dr Panos Barlas)

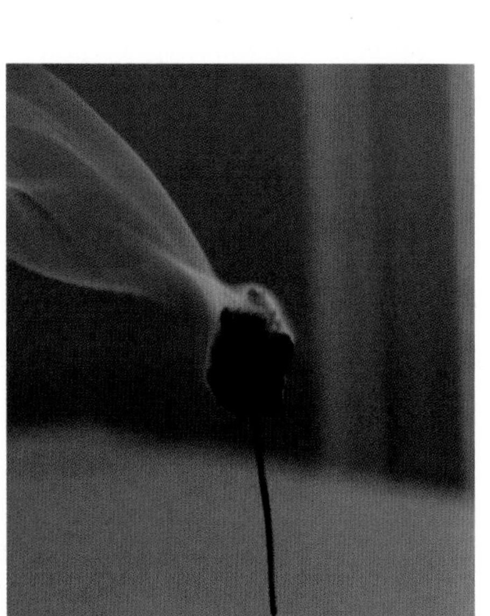

Plate 13 Photograph of moxibustion in the form of a ball of moxa punk pressed around the needle handle and ignited.

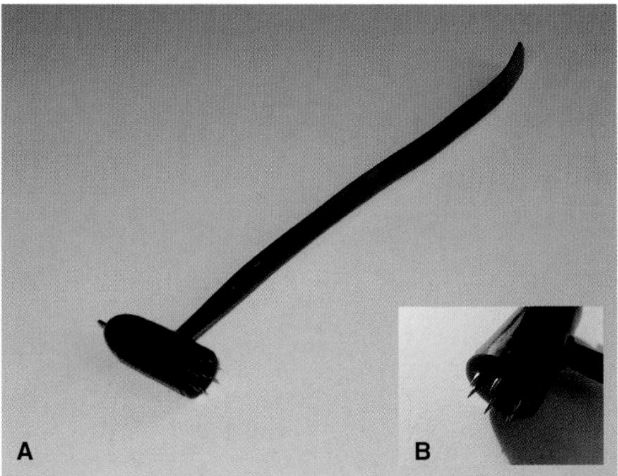

Plate 14 A and B Photograph of 'plum-blossom' needle, showing (A) the whole apparatus and (B) close-up of multiple needles in the head.

headache, etc. (Ezzo et al 2000). The overall results were: weak evidence that acupuncture is superior to inactive controls, such as sham TENS, or to sham acupuncture, such as superficial needling; and inconclusive results when compared with other treatments such as TENS, medication or physiotherapy. This review took careful account of the quality of the studies, and found that the better-quality studies were more likely to be negative – probably because points were awarded for blinding, so higher scoring studies were more likely to use sham acupuncture which, as we have seen, does have some clinical effects.

Dental pain

Although one early review was positive (Ernst & Pittler 1998), it is somewhat difficult to interpret the finding because the studies were varied: the review included both experimental laboratory studies using tooth pain as the outcome, and clinical studies in dental surgery.

Postoperative pain

A large number of studies have tested various forms of acupuncture, given either during or after surgery, for postoperative pain, and many of them show valuable effects in reducing patient-controlled analgesia (Lao et al 1994, Scarsella et al 1994). For example, one study of auricular acupuncture in 54 patients after hip-replacement surgery showed a 30% reduction in pain scores over 3 days (Usichenko et al 2005).

Miscellaneous

For many other painful conditions, including post-herpetic neuralgia and regional pain syndrome, there are insufficient studies to be able to form any conclusions.

Acupuncture for respiratory conditions

Asthma

Eleven studies (324 participants) of acupuncture for asthma have been reviewed (McCarney et al 2004). The evidence is rather confused, according to the reviewers, who comment that the points that were used as active treatment in one trial, based on traditional diagnosis, are used as the inactive control points in other studies. In addition, the reporting of trials was poor and the quality of trials was deemed inadequate to generalize findings, so it is hardly surprising that the reviewers concluded that there was not enough evidence to make any recommendations.

Despite the lack of good-quality evidence, there is continued interest in the use of acupuncture in asthma, particularly by traditional acupuncturists. This may stem from anecdotal reports of dramatic successes in treating asthma. Such reports are merely hypothesis generating; however, they could indicate real effects in a specific subgroup, which are diluted in the RCTs to date. High-quality studies in acute asthma have shown some effect (Fung et al 1986), and it is worth noting that asthma attacks in everyday practice are provoked by a wide range of factors that no single treatment can influence.

From basic science and experimental data, it is conceivable that acupuncture modulates immune function sufficiently in highly responsive individuals to have clinically relevant effects in practice. It is important to remember of course that asthma is a potentially life-threatening disease, and it is critical for patients to continue taking medication to prevent attacks.

Acupuncture for addictions

Smoking cessation

A systematic review of 24 studies of acupuncture and related interventions found that acupuncture was better than doing nothing (one trial). The overall evidence from all studies showed an effect compared with sham acupuncture, but this relied heavily on a single study and disappeared in sensitivity analysis (White et al 2006). Therefore, the conclusions were cautious, i.e. the evidence does not rule an effect in nor rule it out. There is some indirect evidence that continuous acupuncture, using an indwelling stud, may be more effective than other interventions, like hypnotherapy (White & Moody 2006).

Alcohol, heroin and cocaine dependence

Clinical trials into the use of acupuncture for chemical dependence have been weakened by the high dropout rates that are inevitable in this group of patients. This means it is difficult to draw reliable conclusions. Some early studies seemed to show that giving acupuncture according to the NADA protocol (see Chapter 14) reduced the rate at which patients dropped out of the programme. However, recent large studies of 620 patients with heroin or cocaine dependency, or both (Margolin et al 2002) and of 530 patients with alcohol dependency (Bullock et al 2002) found that acupuncture to the 'appropriate' auricular points was no more effective than acupuncture to random control points, or than a relaxation control (Margolin et al 2002) or conventional treatment (Bullock et al 2002) with no acupuncture.

A Cochrane review of auricular acupuncture for cocaine dependency included seven studies with a total of 1433 participants, though not all could be included in the meta-analysis. The review was inconclusive in its overall result (Gates et al 2006).

Trials like these may miss the point of what acupuncture has to offer for drug rehabilitation: the best role of acupuncture may be to calm the drug user when he or she first comes into contact with the drug services, so that they become involved in further care. Anecdotal reports suggest that addicts become relaxed, compliant and positive when they are given acupuncture, and so they become much more willing to involve themselves in treatments such as counselling. Research focused on this specific action of acupuncture has not yet been published.

Acupuncture for central-nervous-system conditions

Stroke

Some of the early studies of acupuncture for stroke rehabilitation were well conducted and rigorous, and suggested there could be a useful effect. For example, when comparing acupuncture with no additional treatment for stroke patients, the quality of life was improved, and patients were much more likely to be at home after 1 year than to be still in hospital or a nursing home (Johansson 1993). Acupuncture seemed to have the potential to save a great deal on costs of rehabilitation. However, subsequent studies of acupuncture against sham treatment seem to show that the effect could have been due simply to expectation or to the additional attention patients received. A meta-analysis of fourteen trials with 1213 patients concluded that, for stroke rehabilitation, acupuncture has no additional effect on motor recovery, but has a small positive effect on disability, which may be due to a true placebo effect (Sze et al 2002). Thus, we are forced to conclude that, although acupuncture is widely used in Eastern countries for stroke patients, the best current evidence suggests that it has no effect beyond placebo.

Acupuncture for nausea and vomiting

Acupuncture treatment for nausea and vomiting is one of the topics that is easiest to research, since patients are plentiful, the treatment standardized (usually PC6 bilaterally) and simple, and any effect is immediate and can be measured in a standardized way. What is not generally agreed yet is whether there is any difference in the effectiveness of treatment with needling, pressure or electrical stimulation.

Nausea of pregnancy

The role of acupuncture in treating nausea in early pregnancy is not completely clear, because the evidence is not uniform. Early studies suggested a powerful effect, but were criticized for being poorly controlled. One rigorous study of acupressure showed no effect compared to either acupressure at an 'inappropriate' point or to no additional treatment (O'Brien et al 1996). One study of acupuncture in 55 women in very early pregnancy found it was not superior to sham treatment using cocktail sticks (Knight et al 2001). A large study with four arms compared full TCM acupuncture with simplified PC6 needling, superficial sham needling and no treatment in 593 women (Smith et al 2002a). All forms of acupuncture were superior to no treatment for nausea (though not for vomiting), with statistical significance at one time or another, but there were no significant differences between the acupuncture groups.

To summarize, the current evidence generally supports the effectiveness of acupressure as a treatment for nausea of pregnancy, but not for vomiting.

Postoperative nausea and vomiting

Twenty-six RCTs (N = 3347) of acupuncture for postoperative nausea and vomiting have been reviewed (Lee & Done 2004). There were significant reductions in nausea, vomiting and the need for rescue antiemetics in the group treated with acupuncture or some other form of stimulation at PC6, compared with the sham treatment group. When compared with antiemetic drugs, there was significant reduction in nausea – but not vomiting – in the PC6 acupoint stimulation group compared with the antiemetic group. However, short-term results were more convincing than the long-term effects. A subsequent review assessed publication bias and concluded that the result for early postoperative vomiting was robust, whereas the result for nausea is less secure and may be affected by unpublished studies (Lee et al 2006).

Nausea and vomiting from chemotherapy

A recent review of 11 trials (N = 1247) found that acupuncture, given in addition to pharmacological antiemetics, reduced the proportion of patients with vomiting, but did not reduce the severity of nausea (Ezzo et al 2005). The effect was more marked with electroacupuncture than with manual acupuncture. Acupressure also seemed effective, but electrical stimulation through surface electrodes was not. The authors were cautious about drawing the conclusion that acupuncture had a place in clinical practice, particularly in comparison with modern pharmacological agents, which are usually very effective.

Acupuncture for genitourinary and reproductive medicine

Gynaecological conditions

For dysmenorrhoea, a review found two trials (N = 62) of acupuncture that demonstrated an effect (White 2003). Two trials of acupressure were also positive.

There are now a number of studies that suggest that acupuncture has a useful effect on postmenopausal hot flushes (Wyon et al 1995, Wyon et al 2004). As is the case with migraine and tension headache, genuine acupuncture appears to have a similar effect to sham acupuncture, but both are superior to no treatment. It is impossible to be sure whether this is because the studies need to be larger to show an effect (type 2 error), or because both forms of treatment have a generalized effect, or because both are only acting through expectation. A large observational study has also shown a prolonged valuable effect of acupuncture on hot flushes in cancer patients (Filshie et al 2005).

Infertility

In the area of infertility, the research so far suggests that acupuncture may have a number of beneficial actions, though the evidence is not conclusive (Stener-Victorin & Humaidan 2006). There is evidence that low-frequency electroacupuncture to the abdominal muscles (with or without stimulation to points in the legs) increases uterine blood flow. Laboratory experiments indicate that the effect is mediated by a supraspinal reflex on the sympathetic innervation (see Chapter 6).

Early results of clinical and laboratory studies suggest that patients with anovulation due to polycystic ovarian syndrome (PCOS) have long-lasting changes from a series of electroacupuncture treatments.

For in-vitro fertilization (IVF), several studies have explored whether acupuncture at the time of embryo transfer has an effect on the pregnancy rate, and the results seem to be positive (Manheimer et al 2008). Both body and auricular acupuncture for infertility, compared with usual care, were positive, though one study used acupuncture specifically for analgesia during oocyte aspiration.

Acupuncture in pregnancy

The effects of acupuncture on pelvic pain and back pain and on nausea in pregnancy are reviewed in the relevant sections above.

Acupuncture seems to be useful in reducing labour pain according to three trials summarized in a recent review (Lee & Ernst 2004). A large observational study of nearly 18 000 women found that the patients who chose acupuncture during labour were less likely to require epidural analgesia (Nesheim & Kinge 2006). There is also some evidence that acupuncture ripens the cervix at term and shortens labour (Gaudernack et al 2006).

Urological conditions

For women with irritative bladder (urgency, urge incontinence, frequency and nocturia), an RCT in 39 women showed that acupuncture is as effective as treatment with the standard anticholinergic drug oxybutinin, with significantly fewer adverse events and, as a result, significantly fewer dropouts (Kelleher et al 1994).

An RCT in 100 women with recurrent urinary infection found that following acupuncture treatment, 73% of women who received acupuncture were free from infection compared with 52% of the control group who had no treatment; the difference just failed to meet statistical significance (Alraek et al 2002). One subgroup with a particular type of history seemed to fare better (Alraek & Baerheim 2003).

Miscellaneous

Skin conditions

A recent RCT comparing acupuncture with sham acupuncture in 40 patients with uraemic pruritus suggests that acupuncture is significantly superior (Chou et al 2005, also referenced as Cheh-Yi C).

Tinnitus

A review of controlled trials included two open studies and four sham controlled trials in 185 patients (Park et al 2000). Four of the studies were of crossover design, which might introduce problems because patients may notice the difference between the treatments in the two arms. In addition, in one study a patient responded completely to acupuncture in the first arm and, therefore, withdrew – which actually biases the results against acupuncture. A careful reading of the studies indicates that acupuncture might be useful in some individual patients. The review concluded overall that there was no convincing evidence that acupuncture has an effect on tinnitus, and this finding is supported by a large ($N = 300$) controlled trial from Sweden (Cummings & Lundeberg 2006). The authors conclude that cognitive-behavioural therapy should be offered before acupuncture.

The cost effectiveness of acupuncture

Several doctors practising acupuncture in primary care in the UK have conducted studies that have shown how acupuncture might save money for the National Health Service. Myers et al found that patients given acupuncture used smaller amounts of analgesic and anti-inflammatory drugs during the following 6 months (Myers 1991). Lindall measured the costs of a properly funded acupuncture clinic, and estimated that it would have saved money by reducing referral to (more expensive) secondary care clinics (Lindall 1999). Ross showed that the number of referrals to physiotherapy and to rheumatology outpatients fell by 86% and by 51%, respectively, over the 3 years during which she was incorporating acupuncture practice into her daily surgery (Ross 2001).

Rigorous evaluation of the economic aspects of treatments depends on careful measurement of the actual cost of treatment in relation to the improvement in patients' health. The patients' health is assessed by a standard measure called the QALY (Quality Adjusted Life Year), which takes into account both the prolongation of life (if any) in years, and the quality of life during that time, on a scale of zero (dead) to one (in complete health). This measure operates in the same way for all treatments in all conditions and, thus, allows a true comparison of the cost effectiveness of different treatments. Now, acupuncture does not extend life in any condition (except, arguably, in smoking cessation), so its effects are measured solely by the increase in quality of life as a result of treatment. When acupuncture is compared with usual care, the comparison is known as the ICER (incremental cost effectiveness ratio): this measures the cost of improving the patients' health with acupuncture. The units are '£ per QALY'. In the UK, The National Institute for Health and Clinical Excellence (NICE) use ICERs to evaluate the place of new treatments, and as a general rule will recommend treatments that cost less than £20 000 per QALY, and may recommend treatments costing more £ per QALY, depending on other criteria.

The economic analyses of acupuncture that have been performed and published at this date are summarized in Table 9.1. Consider the two studies performed in the UK: for back pain, acupuncture treatment cost in the region of £200 per patient (Ratcliffe et al 2006); this cost was slightly offset by lower use of other healthcare services (including pain clinic) over the trial period and the overall ICER (cost per QALY) was £4241. For chronic headache, the cost effectiveness of acupuncture was estimated at £9180 per QALY (Wonderling et al 2004). Both these estimates are competitive when compared to many accepted medical interventions.

The main cost of an acupuncture service is the cost of the acupuncturist, including the overheads, such as professional development and management

TABLE 9.1

The cost effectiveness of acupuncture, from full economic evaluations of randomized controlled trials

Condition	Number *N* =	Context	Follow-up	Cost per Quality Adjusted Life Year
Back pain (Ratcliffe et al 2006)	241	Private acupuncturist	2 years	£4241
Back pain (Witt et al 2006c)	2388	Physician acupuncturist[a]	6 months	£7157
Headache (Wonderling et al 2004)	401	Private physiotherapist	1 year	£9180
Headache (Witt et al 2006a)	2682	Physician acupuncturist	3 months	£7881
Neck pain (Witt et al 2006a)	3005	Physician acupuncturist[a]	3 months	£8479
Osteoarthritis knee or hip (Witt et al 2006a)	421	Physician acupuncturist[a]	3 months	£12 135

[a]Conducted in Germany, ICER in euro converted to sterling at €1 = £0.68 (2007 rate). Other studies conducted in the UK.

of the service. In reality, resourceful practitioners will find ways of reducing these costs to a minimum in order to be able to provide a valuable service to their patients. Many GPs and physiotherapists and other healthcare workers who are already employed in the health service manage to incorporate acupuncture into their everyday practice without diminishing the care of other patients. Another option is to organize the service so that several patients can be treated at the same time. This kind of arrangement can significantly improve the cost effectiveness of acupuncture, and is well worth investigating as a means of delivering acupuncture effectively in a resource-limited health service.

At the Royal London Homoeopathic Hospital, a senior nurse trained in acupuncture currently provides formula electroacupuncture for osteoarthritis of the knee, treating up to 12 patients each hour in a 'high volume clinic'. The clinical effects shown in an audit of the results seem to be in line with those of the large RCTs.

Summary

There are a number of difficulties in designing rigorous clinical trails of acupuncture, such as the lack of suitable inert placebo control, difficulties blinding the practitioner, knowing what conditions to investigate, and lack of research capacity and resources to pursue a logical and totally thorough research pathway. In addition, acupuncture is a complex intervention and needs an imaginative approach.

Studies have repeatedly shown that acupuncture is more effective than doing nothing for many conditions, and has an effect large enough to be clinically useful. The strongest evidence that acupuncture is superior to placebo is for postoperative nausea, chronic knee pain and low back pain. There is a trend for the newer systematic reviews to produce more positive results when they incorporate the modern, more rigorous and better designed studies. In many clinical areas, however, the evidence that acupuncture has a valuable clinical effect relies more on common sense interpretation of observational studies and case series than on sham-controlled clinical trials.

CHAPTER

10

Evidence on the safety of acupuncture

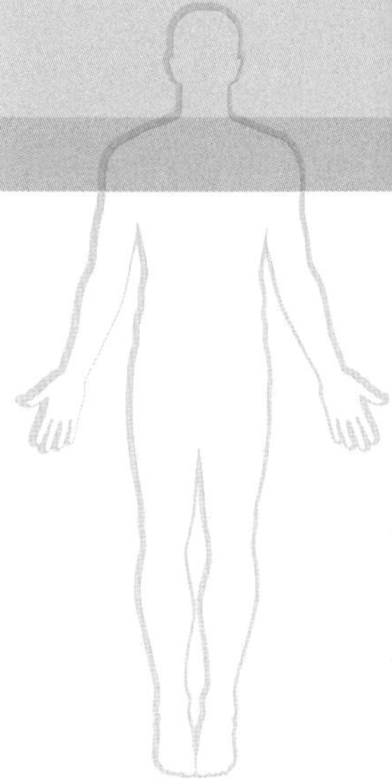

Contents

After reading this chapter, you should be able to:

- name four common mild adverse events of acupuncture
- name one unavoidable adverse event
- name three serious adverse events.

Introduction: acupuncture is safe in skilled hands

Acupuncture has a reputation for safety, and this has now been confirmed by a number of prospective surveys in different countries.

In one survey between 1998 and 2000, 78 doctors and physiotherapists in the UK reported adverse events that occurred during or after 32 000 consultations involving acupuncture (White et al 2001). No serious adverse events were reported and minor events, such as bleeding, occurred on average in less than 7% of treatments. These figures are essentially similar to the findings of other studies among trained practitioners and in a variety of countries, such as a survey of 34 000 treatments by 1848 non-medical acupuncturists over a 4-week period in the UK (MacPherson et al 2001); a survey of over 65 000 treatments given in a Japanese acupuncture clinic – which found nothing more serious to report than nine cases in which a needle was not removed at the end of treatment (Yamashita et al 1999); and a survey of 3535 acupuncture treatments by 29 doctors and other health professionals in Germany (Ernst et al 2003). An editorial in the *British Medical Journal* that reviewed the evidence from these various surveys summarized the situation thus: 'Acupuncture ... certainly seems, in skilled hands, one of the safer forms of medical intervention' (Vincent 2001).

One of the strengths of the safety record of acupuncture is that, since it is mainly used to treat musculoskeletal pain, it is replacing drugs such as non-steroidal anti-inflammatory drugs (NSAIDs). These have several major side effects, particularly upper-gastrointestinal bleeding or perforation, increasing the risk of this by a factor of about four (Hernandez-Diaz & Rodriguez 2000), as well as causing renal damage, hypertension and increased risk of stroke.

The evidence on safety of acupuncture is not as straightforward as it may appear from the overall picture given by the surveys, however. Their results showed that there is wide variation in the rate of adverse events reported by different practitioners. For example, one practitioner reported bleeding in 53% of patients after acupuncture, whereas others reported no bleeding at all. Some of this variation will be due to differences in reporting – practitioners who tend to be very cautious are likely to report every small bleeding event, even though the survey's intention was to record only significant amounts of bleeding. Also, some of the variation between individual practitioners may be due to differences between their types of patient (for example, a practice consisting of elderly patients might expect more bleeding because they may have more fragile vessels and less subcutaneous tissue); and some may be due to different styles of acupuncture. But it also seems likely that adverse events do vary with the technique and skill of the practitioner. It is obviously not enough for a practitioner to simply think 'acupuncture is safe'; each has the responsibility to think constantly about safety to ensure that the adverse event rate is as low as possible.

Detailed recommendations for the safe practice of acupuncture are given in Chapter 13, and in this chapter we are concentrating solely on a discussion of the published evidence. Knowing what has happened before helps us to avoid doing the same.

Apart from problems from the needling, there is another potential source of risk to patients from acupuncture: they may miss out on conventional treatment that would have been more effective for their condition. This so-called '*indirect*' risk can obviously be serious, for example, if patients are not given the chance of an early diagnosis of their cancer because their symptoms are not interpreted correctly. This book is written in the assumption that every patient considered for acupuncture will have undergone a conventional medical diagnosis, and will have been informed when conventional treatment would give a better likelihood of recovery than acupuncture can offer.

A modern approach to safety

The prevailing attitude to safety in many healthcare services now promotes improvements in practice, but sometimes appears to concentrate on finding the 'guilty' individual. We should be looking instead for guilty systems that let the accident occur. But it is not just the authorities that need to change attitude. After an adverse event, doctors who regard themselves as 'responsible' may experience considerable self-recrimination. Medical students have been imbued with the concept of the Hippocratic oath, which is understood to mean 'first do no harm'; and so injuring a patient through an 'error' seems to be the antithesis of their vocation.

Patients who complain after a medical injury are not usually seeking compensation and are more interested in ensuring that the mistake does not happen to other patients. However, the blame culture tends to make the event more likely to be covered up, for fear and embarrassment and to avoid legal consequences. A common feeling among colleagues and other professionals is, 'Thank goodness it wasn't me', rather than, 'What were the underlying causes?'. Any enquiry will probably concentrate on the actions of the practitioners immediately before the event, rather than looking for failures in the background circumstances which allowed it to happen.

A totally different approach to accidents has been developed in commercial flying, another profession where errors can be disastrous, and this is recommended as a model for the health professions. The positive approach to safety recognizes that errors are inevitable; we should aim to reduce them by identifying the *systems* failure that allowed or encouraged errors to take place – not the individual. Every incident is regarded as an opportunity to learn significant lessons and a stimulus to incorporate them into practice throughout the whole of the profession.

Accidents in acupuncture are often the end result of several coinciding difficulties: problems such as pressure of work, professional isolation, lack of learning and updating knowledge of anatomy, and difficult working conditions such as poor lighting.

> *Wise men learn by other men's mistakes; fools learn by their own.*
>
> *(Anon)*

We encourage readers to use this review of the adverse events, and the comments on safe practice in Chapter 13, to formulate a considered and reflective approach to safety; safety should be an integral part of learning acupuncture, and should be continually reinforced. Safe practice depends on establishing safe attitudes and systems in at least these areas:

- Learning, both initially and continuously
- Protocols and procedures
- Equipment
- Practice organization
- Physical and mental health including effects of stress and motivation
- Attitude and support from professional colleagues
- Regulation.

The potential risks of acupuncture

It is useful to discuss adverse events in three degrees of severity, shown in Table 10.1.

TABLE 10.1

A classification of mild, significant and serious adverse events, as used in this chapter

Severity	Definition
Mild	Reversible, short lived and does not seriously inconvenience the patient
Significant	Needs medical attention or interferes with the patient's normal activities
Serious	Requires hospital admission or prolongation of existing hospital stay, or results in persistent or significant disability/incapacity or death

It is not easy to obtain reliable figures about the rates of risk in acupuncture, because there are inevitably biases and inaccuracies in reporting: adverse events may be under-reported by patients because they do not want to upset their practitioner; they are under-reported by the acupuncturist who may not be aware of the ethical need to describe such events; but over-reported by other health professionals who dislike acupuncture for some reason and wish to damage its reputation.

Also, *attribution* of any event to acupuncture treatment may not be straightforward: it may be difficult to know whether an event was caused by acupuncture or not. There are standard methods of attributing cause, including the time relationship of onset and offset, biomedical rationale, and repeated sequelae on re-exposure. However, in individual cases, especially the more serious and complex ones, several events may contribute to the outcome and the precise contribution of different causes cannot be accurately deduced.

The figures for the rates of adverse events given here are based on the published evidence, but should be regarded as only an approximation. Anyway, our main interest is practical, so learning how we can make acupuncture practice safer is a major objective in this book.

Mild events

The most common events during or after acupuncture, with typical incidence rates (expressed as a per cent of treatments), are:

- bleeding, more than a small drop: about 3%
- aggravation of symptoms: about 1–2%
- needling pain, more than a little sharpness: about 1%
- drowsiness: up to about 1%
- faintness: usually less than 0.5%.

This rate of minor adverse events is low enough to be officially classed as 'minimal'. Other events that are less commonly reported include nausea and headache. These figures are those reported by practitioners: patients tend to have a lower threshold for identifying symptoms, and so they report higher rates. For example, in one series patients reported that they found 13% of needle insertions painful, and that they were drowsy after 8% of sessions (Yamashita et al 2000).

Mild adverse events are reported in about 3% of acupuncture treatments.

Two minor events – aggravation of symptoms, and drowsiness – need further comment. Some practitioners argue that acupuncture is a 'natural' treatment, it is inevitable that it will make problems worse before they improve, and so any aggravation of symptoms is an acceptable part of 'the healing response'. This idea may reassure patients, but there is no evidence that it is true. In one study in which the incidence of aggravation was recorded together with the eventual outcome, aggravation was not followed by a better response to treatment; the rate of success in patients is about 70%, with or without aggravation. Plenty of patients respond to treatment without getting worse first. This all suggests that aggravation may not, in fact, be necessary for a response to acupuncture, and we, therefore, recommend that practitioners should take care to avoid aggravation, particularly by not using too strong a treatment at the first session.

Relaxation is often regarded as a benefit of treatment: but drowsiness can be serious enough to increase the danger posed by anyone who is driving or using machinery. In one study, about one-third of patients experienced some degree of drowsiness (Brattberg 1986), and only slightly less in a recent study (MacPherson & Thomas 2005).

Significant events

Skin infections that need treatment have been reported on a number of occasions. These generally involve the typical opportunistic commensal bacteria, but four cases of infection with *Mycobacterium* have been reported. Cases of cellulitis have occurred when acupuncture needles were inserted into areas of oedema. Occasionally, acupuncture seems to reactivate herpes zoster infection.

Peripheral nerve injury from acupuncture has been reported on a few occasions leading to, for example, foot drop. The question arises as to why this kind of nerve injury is not reported more often when acupuncture needles must penetrate nerves quite frequently? The usual explanation given is that acupuncture needles have non-cutting tips, which push the nerve fibres apart.

Exacerbation of asthma is not uncommon during or after treatment, and may be serious enough to require hospital admission. Seizures can occur in patients who faint because they are treated sitting up (which is not recommended, for this reason). Very occasionally, a seizure occurs in a patient who is lying down: here the diagnosis may be reflex anoxic seizure due to a marked vagal response to needling, involving the limbic system.

Other kinds of major collapse during acupuncture are rare, but some have been reported. A few patients have been reported to simply go unconscious, either when the needles are inserted or when they are stimulated. There is no associated cardiovascular collapse, so the mechanism must be purely neurological. If not already supine, such patients need to be laid down immediately. Fortunately it is extremely rare and the patients recover completely.

Serious events

These can best be considered under the headings of traumatic and infectious. Tables 10.2 and 10.3 show the cases described in 'primary' reports, i.e.

TABLE 10.2

Serious traumatic events reported in association with acupuncture

Condition or organ	Number reported	Comment
Lung and pleurae	54	Pneumothorax, one haemothorax
Heart and pericardium	9	Mostly cardiac tamponade
Blood vessels	10	Includes compartment syndrome, deep vein thrombosis, popliteal artery occlusion, and pseudoaneurysm
Brain, spinal cord	12	Mostly penetration of the medulla or brainstem from needling the upper neck posteriorly; also, two cases of transverse myelopathy from spinal cord trauma

TABLE 10.3

Serious infections reported in association with acupuncture

Infection	Number reported	Comment
Hepatitis B	148	Reuse of needles
HIV	4	Reuse of needles
Auricular chondritis	14	
Endocarditis	6	
Meningitis	1	
Spinal infection	3	Two spinal, one epidural
Septicaemia	5	
Necrotizing fasciitis and toxic shock	3	
Septic arthritis	3	Shoulder, knee and sacroiliac joints
Abscess	7	Abdomen, neck, psoas muscle, other retroperitoneal site, soft tissue and temporomandibular joint
Other reported	4	Include infected compartment, infected eyeball, osteomyelitis

reports written by a practitioner directly involved in the case (White 2004). There are also a roughly similar number of 'secondary' reports, i.e. written by someone who did not witness the case. These are obviously less reliable and so are not considered in detail here.

In interpreting these tables, it is important to remember the difficulties of accurate attribution mentioned above. It is also important to recognize that the great majority of traumatic events can be avoided by applying a good knowledge of anatomy, and the great majority of infectious events avoided by good hygiene and the use of sterile equipment.

Serious adverse events can be almost completely eliminated by good practice.

A number of deaths have been reported in association with acupuncture, which we summarize to draw attention to the main risks of acupuncture. We are aware of 12 primary reports and 39 secondary reports. The deaths could not be attributed to acupuncture 'for certain' in all cases. Of the primary reports, six were traumatic, of which four were due to pneumothorax and two to cardiac tamponade. One of the tamponade cases was an 82-year-old woman who gave herself acupuncture with a sewing needle. Five deaths were due to infection, including two from septicaemia, and one each of hepatitis, pyohaemothorax and toxic shock syndrome. The twelfth death was from an acute asthma attack: the patient had acupuncture for the attack, but failed to respond. This case emphasizes the need not to rely on acupuncture alone to treat serious conditions, and not to abandon the conventional management with drugs.

The secondary reports are in the Chinese literature, and include 13 deaths from pneumothorax, nine from cardiac or aortic injury, eight from injury to the central nervous system (CNS) (seven to the medulla, one to the cerebellum), and three from trauma to the liver (Huang 1996). One case was reported to have been due to laryngeal spasm, and in five cases no details were available. Seven of these deaths were reported to be after treatment by unqualified practitioners. In some cases needles had been inserted through clothing.

The overall risk of serious adverse events associated with acupuncture can be estimated from the evidence of 13 prospective studies involving over four million treatments that reported 11 events, none of which was fatal (White 2006). The cumulative worldwide rate for serious adverse events with acupuncture is, therefore, estimated to be 0.02 per 10 000 treatments, which represents 'negligible' risk, well below that of most medical treatments.

Overall, acupuncture presents a 'negligible' risk of adverse events.

Unavoidable events

There is no doubt that some reactions to acupuncture are unavoidable, in that they are inevitable in individual patients, but cannot be predicted. These reactions are described in every survey, even those of Japanese acupuncture where needles are generally inserted very superficially into the subcutaneous layer only. The most serious of these is severe drowsiness, which may constitute a real risk of road traffic accidents. Clearly some patients are more susceptible than others. The decision on whether to give acupuncture to such patients again depends on a risk–benefit assessment: the same reaction is likely to recur on further treatment, though drowsiness is one reaction that generally becomes less severe when the treatment is repeated.

Drowsiness after acupuncture can be serious: patients must be advised how to manage it.

Indirect risk

The risk from acupuncture is described as 'indirect' if the harm is caused by the practitioner rather than the practice. This would usually be when a patient does not receive more appropriate treatment because the practitioner made an incorrect diagnosis, or believed acupuncture to be more effective than it is in this case, or was not aware of the evidence that acupuncture is less effective than other treatment.

Summary

Acupuncture is generally safe in skilled hands, as shown by the evidence from several prospective surveys. One of acupuncture's strengths is its safety compared with other treatments.

Acupuncture does carry some risks – traumatic, infectious and miscellaneous. Also acupuncture can be a source of 'indirect' risk if it is used instead of another more effective treatment. The rates of adverse events vary from practitioner to practitioner, and each has a responsibility to develop and maintain safe practice. A non-blaming approach to safety seeks to examine and improve the systems around the practitioner, including training, procedures and protocols and practice organization.

The most common mild adverse events after acupuncture are bleeding, pain on needling and aggravation of symptoms, followed by faintness and drowsiness (which may affect driving). Significant events are less common and include skin infections, peripheral nerve injury, exacerbations of asthma and seizure. Serious events are very rare, but include cardiac tamponade, injury to blood vessels or central nervous tissue, and infections such as hepatitis B, endocarditis and auricular chondritis. Some side effects are unavoidable. Overall, the risk of adverse events from acupuncture is 'negligible'.

SECTION 3 PRACTICAL ASPECTS

Preparation for treatment

CHAPTER

11

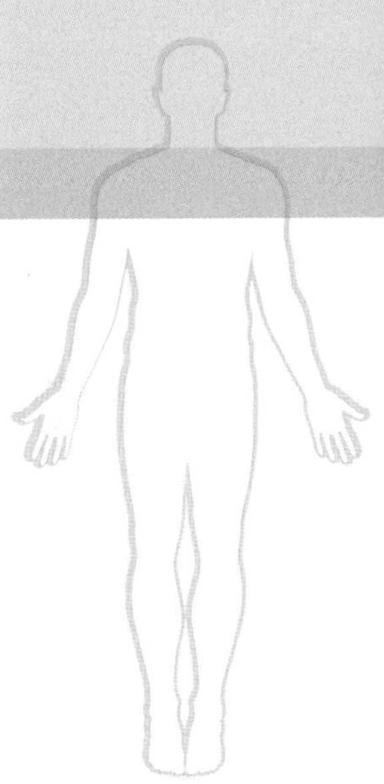

Contents

After reading this chapter you should be able to:

- state two absolute contraindications to acupuncture
- state one contraindication to indwelling needles
- state four relative contraindications to acupuncture
- state four conditions requiring special precautions
- state the diameter and length of a standard needle.

Introduction

Acupuncture is in some senses a straightforward matter of inserting a few needles, but for treatment to be safe and effective, some preparation is necessary. It is particularly important for beginners to establish good habits and routines as soon as they start practice. Safety, just as much as effectiveness, must become second nature when treating patients.

As well as ensuring that they have the best training and continued education, acupuncturists should apply the standards expected of all healthcare professionals: they should conduct themselves at all times in a suitable manner. An example of appropriate behaviour and ethical standards is given in the various documents that make up the General Medical Council's *Good Medical Practice*.

One aspect of good patient care is that there is appropriate communication between all the practitioners involved in the patient's care. Acupuncturists who work independently should try to ensure (with the patient's permission), that the patient's GP knows that they are seeing the patient, both for clinical and for ethical reasons.

Practitioners must have a realistic and honest approach to what the acupuncture can achieve. Claims that acupuncture can treat anything and everything are false, deceive patients, and bring the therapy into disrepute. Claims for magical cures are short-sighted: acupuncture is a form of therapy with successes and failures, like most treatments.

This chapter describes the thinking processes behind safe and effective acupuncture, up to the moment of inserting the needles. This is the preparation for the treatment itself, which is described in the following chapter. This chapter has not been designed to be used as the basis for formal guidelines for providing services, and readers who need to develop guidelines could base them on an example written for palliative care (Filshie & Hester 2006).

Patients suitable for acupuncture

Patients for acupuncture should be screened for possible contraindications and for the need for special precautions.

Contraindications

The patient must be willing to receive acupuncture. There are two main reasons why the patient might not be willing:

1. Needle phobia
2. Personal belief: occasionally, patients believe that acupuncture, because it is associated with ideas of energy and meridians, can have an adverse spiritual influence, so they want nothing to do with it. It is tempting to try to circumvent these beliefs by using some phrase like 'dry needling', but probably not sensible. We prefer to mention the word 'acupuncture', and let the patient decide.

A tiny proportion of the population can react to an invasive medical technique by having a convulsion; the mechanism is not clear, but may involve a sudden strong vagal stimulus to the heart. The significance of this reaction is that it cannot necessarily be avoided by treatment with the patient lying flat. This should not be confused with the sort of mild anoxic convulsion that can occur if a patient faints and cannot immediately be lain down flat. If there is a history of an unexplained convulsion prior to a patient presenting for acupuncture, it is wise to avoid acupuncture treatment. Inevitably, some patients with this reaction will receive acupuncture as their first medical intervention, in which case such events should be regarded as unavoidable.

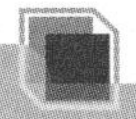

BOX 11.1

Contraindications for acupuncture

ABSOLUTE CONTRAINDICATIONS TO ACUPUNCTURE

- Patient unwilling
- Spontaneous bleeding or bruising (unless fully assessed).

ABSOLUTE CONTRAINDICATIONS TO A PARTICULAR TECHNIQUE

- Valvular heart disease: avoid indwelling needles
- Demand-type pacemaker, or intracardiac defibrillator: avoid electroacupuncture across the chest.

RELATIVE CONTRAINDICATIONS

- Severe bleeding tendency, e.g. anticoagulant therapy, thrombocytopenia
- Psychologically disturbed patients (may have unpredictable reactions)
- Compromised immune system
- Previous seizure induced by an invasive medical procedure
- Marked previous reaction to acupuncture.

Patients who bruise spontaneously should not be treated until their clotting function has been checked and is satisfactory.

These contraindications are listed in Box 11.1.

Absolute contraindications to particular techniques

- Indwelling needles are a potential source for bacteraemia, which can infect a damaged heart causing subacute bacterial endocarditis. (High risk: previous endocarditis, previous cardiac surgery including valve prosthesis and congenital valvular disease, such as Marfan's syndrome; low risk: rheumatic heart disease, calcified aortic valve and floppy mitral valve.)
- Electrical stimulation may possibly affect the sensing mechanism of a pacemaker or intracardiac defibrillator.

Relative contraindications: balancing risk and benefit

A patient may have a 'relative' contraindication to acupuncture. In this case, it is the practitioner's responsibility to work with the patient in striking a balance between the benefits and risks of treatment. For example, faced with a patient with a bleeding disorder due to anticoagulant drugs, you may decide not to use deep needling for treating ankylosing spondylitis: the expectation of benefit is small, and deep needling runs a significant risk of causing haemorrhage. On the other hand, you might use superficial needling, which could be safe and effective for a patient with tension headache. Take the patient's views into account, but do not allow a patient to persuade you to give treatment when you believe it is contraindicated.

Special precautions

This section deals with precautions that can be anticipated from the condition of the patient (Box 11.2). There are additional precautions that are necessary due to local conditions at the point, which will be discussed in the following chapter.

Patients with a bleeding tendency

A bleeding tendency due to conditions such as haemophilia, thrombocytopenia or taking anticoagulant drugs is a 'relative contraindication', but if you decide to treat the patient then you should take special precautions. It might be hard to justify needling patients who have extremely low platelet counts, for example, but acupuncture may be a useful alternative for patients with moderate bleeding disorder (Box 11.3).

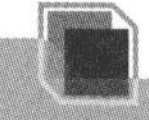

BOX 11.2

Cases where special precautions are required in using acupuncture

SPECIAL PRECAUTIONS

- Bleeding tendency (see text)
- Epilepsy: do not leave the patient unattended
- Immunosuppression, whether due to medical condition or drug treatment: extra attention to hygiene
- Pregnancy (see text)
- Patient without a clear diagnosis: acupuncture may mask symptoms of serious conditions such as cancer, delaying diagnosis
- Abnormal physical structure: increased risk of trauma, especially if underweight
- Patient who needs to drive after acupuncture treatment: treat lightly, rest and observe after treatment and advise to stop driving if drowsy
- Strong reactors to acupuncture (see text).

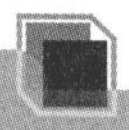

BOX 11.3

Acupuncture used in a patient with thrombocytopenia

A 39-year-old woman developed thrombocytopenia in her second pregnancy. She had a caesarean section under general anaesthetic, since spinal and epidural anaesthesia were contraindicated by her platelet count of 82×10^9/l. In the postoperative phase, standard analgesic drugs did not provide sufficient pain relief, but acupuncture had a rapid, useful effect, without causing excessive bleeding (Oomman et al 2005).

In patients with a bleeding tendency, acupuncture should be performed with particular care:

- Consider using fine needles, perhaps with electrical stimulation for the less sensitive patients.
- Avoid deep or vigorous needling in the enclosed fascial compartments of the lower limbs and forearms, because of the potential risk of compartment syndrome.
- Take particular care when needling near joints, because of the increased risk of haemarthrosis.
- Apply firm pressure to points after removing the needles.

Pregnancy

Many acupuncture teachers advise their students to use acupuncture carefully, if at all, in the first trimester of pregnancy on the grounds that 'it may cause a spontaneous abortion'. However, even at full term there is little evidence that acupuncture can induce labour. Acupuncture is frequently used in China to treat many conditions in the first trimester of pregnancy without applying any special precautions. Its use in early pregnancy is also clearly established in the West for treating nausea.

Acupuncturists who are nervous of litigation will argue: 'Even if you don't cause an abortion, you may be blamed if one occurs within a few days of your acupuncture session'. This is defensive medicine, which often does not lead to good treatment. There is now some evidence from a controlled trial involving 593 women with nausea of pregnancy that the outcomes of pregnancy (both pregnancy outcomes and health of child) are not affected by acupuncture (Smith et al 2002b). We suggest that:

- acupuncture can be used throughout pregnancy
- risks and the benefits of treatment are weighed in the usual way
- in the first trimester, it is probably wise to avoid strong stimulation techniques.

Strong reactors

Some patients react strongly to acupuncture: when given normal strength treatment, they are more than usually likely to experience:

- aggravation of their symptoms
- feelings of fatigue immediately after treatment
- feelings of malaise after treatment, sometimes amounting to an influenza-like syndrome for 2 or 3 days.

About 5–10% of a primary care population will have a reaction to a dose of treatment that has no adverse effect on the remaining 90–95%, but the rate is higher in cancer patients.

It is difficult to judge a patient's sensitivity in advance. Felix Mann observed that artistic types and those who have a strongly charitable outlook are more likely to be strong reactors. Sometimes a patient will give a clue in that a previous physical treatment – massage or manipulation for example – produced an unpleasant reaction. In that case it is best to assume that acupuncture will do the same.

Fortunately, strong *reactors* are also usually good *responders*. These patients have a strong therapeutic response, so treatment can be light: in the most sensitive patients, as little as 30 seconds' needling may be enough.

Similarly, children in general are likely to be strong reactors and the needle should be removed within a few seconds. However, unlike adults, this does not mean that all children are good responders.

Patients with cancer

Acupuncture can be very helpful for the palliation of symptoms in cancer patients, but special precautions are required for many reasons, including the facts that these patients may have significant side effects of their treatment and even multi-organ disease. There is a risk of masking symptoms, and a need to recognize that a patient who fails to respond to treatment in the usual way may have an increased tumour load. A fuller discussion of these issues is available for anyone who wishes to treat these patients (Filshie 2001).

Information and informed consent

Patients must be given adequate information about the benefits and risks of acupuncture to allow them to make a fully informed decision about treatment. The difficulty is in knowing what is meant by 'adequate' information, but it should include an offer of:

- realistic information about the possible expected benefits of acupuncture
- information about the known risks of acupuncture relevant to the case
- other available treatments for the condition, if relevant.

It is obviously important to strike a balance between, on the one hand, not concealing risks that are real and relevant and, on the other hand, officiously listing every adverse event that has ever been associated with acupuncture. This could frighten patients away from using a treatment that might benefit them.

All information about risk must be given in plain language that is appropriate for the individual patient; and you should judge (and ideally justify) when individual patients have gained the information they need and want. Patients should also be offered information about the risks and benefits of any other treatment available. It would be unethical to recommend acupuncture for a condition when there is no convincing evidence that it is effective, but when some other treatment is known to be effective. Patients must be informed and then make their own decision.

Normally, verbal consent to treatment is enough. Some hospital trusts or other employers of acupuncturists may insist on providing written information and sometimes obtaining signed consent. The patient information leaflet reproduced here (Box 11.4) was developed by consent between several UK

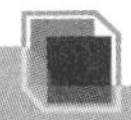

BOX 11.4

Patient information sheet and consent form

Please read this information carefully, and ask your practitioner if there is anything that you do not understand.

WHAT IS ACUPUNCTURE?

Acupuncture is a form of therapy in which fine needles are inserted into specific points on the body.

IS ACUPUNCTURE SAFE?

Acupuncture is generally very safe. Serious side effects are very rare – less than one per 10 000 treatments.

DOES ACUPUNCTURE HAVE SIDE EFFECTS?

You need to be aware that:

- drowsiness occurs after treatment in a small number of patients, and, if affected, you are advised not to drive
- minor bleeding or bruising occurs after acupuncture in about 3% of treatments
- pain during treatment occurs in about 1% of treatments
- symptoms can get worse after treatment (less than 3% of patients). You should tell your acupuncturist about this, but it is usually a good sign
- fainting can occur in certain patients, particularly at the first treatment.

In addition, if there are particular risks that apply in your case, your practitioner will discuss these with you.

IS THERE ANYTHING YOUR PRACTITIONER NEEDS TO KNOW?

Apart from the usual medical details, it is important that you let your practitioner know:

- if you have ever experienced a fit, faint or funny turn
- if you have a pacemaker or any other electrical implants
- if you have a bleeding disorder
- if you are taking anticoagulants or any other medication
- if you have damaged heart valves or have any other particular risk of infection.

Single-use, sterile, disposable needles are used in the clinic.

STATEMENT OF CONSENT

I confirm that I have read and understood the above information, and I consent to having acupuncture treatment. I understand that I can refuse treatment at any time.

Signature

Print name in full

Date

acupuncture professional organizations. It includes an optional space for patient consent, but a signature is less important, legally speaking, than making sure that patients are satisfied that they have enough information to make a decision. Practitioners who wish to use the form in their own practice may download it from http://www.medical-acupuncture.co.uk/journal/2001(2)/page_123.pdf

In fact, patients are considered to have given consent *for the examination* by preparing themselves, i.e. by undressing or by climbing on the couch, after being given adequate information. It might be natural to assume that this consent includes having treatment, but be aware that further consent may be needed because:

- patients may be willing to be examined, but want to reserve the right to decide on treatment after the examination
- you may not be able to predict the possible benefits of treatment until you have examined the patient, in which case you should provide this information then.

Also, if you have been using manual acupuncture and want to introduce electroacupuncture, it is worth discussing this with the patient, if electroacupuncture was not expressly included in your initial discussion about acupuncture.

Conditions suitable for acupuncture

Acupuncture is most often used for various musculoskeletal problems (Table 11.1). Myofascial trigger point pain seems to respond quickest and best, followed by other soft-tissue injuries that have been slow to heal, followed by osteoarthritis. Acupuncturists disagree amongst themselves about which conditions respond best, because their opinions are formed by anecdotes of particular patients they remember doing well or badly, and because a practitioner's particular interest in a condition might improve his skill and influence his approach and raise expectations.

Acupuncture will not reverse structural changes, like the degeneration of joint surfaces in osteoarthritis, though it can still give symptom relief and reduce inflammation. This fact may be obvious to the practitioner, but should be made explicit to the patient who may misunderstand what friends have told them and may come for acupuncture believing, for example, that it will heal their arthritic joints.

The patient's history may suggest that the symptoms could be due either to underlying pathology or to myofascial trigger points (MTrPs) imitating the condition. It may be difficult to be sure clinically since MTrPs could be present in both cases. Patients respond to acupuncture better when the symptoms are caused primarily by trigger points. For example, dysmenorrhoea due to endometriosis is unlikely to be helped much by acupuncture, but similar symptoms from trigger points in the abdominal wall are likely to respond.

Nociceptive pain responds more reliably than neurogenic pain or pain of no known cause, and acupuncture for these conditions should be regarded as a kind of therapeutic trial.

Like many other therapies, acupuncture works best on earlier and milder cases, before the disease pattern becomes thoroughly ingrained and complicated with psychological changes.

TABLE 11.1

Some common conditions for which patients request acupuncture, and a general indication of the likelihood of a useful clinical response

Response likely	Response possible: moderate or limited cases	Response unlikely: rare or idiosyncratic
Musculoskeletal conditions		
Trigger point pain (myofascial) Osteoarthritis (especially knee, ankle, acromio-clavicular joint, cervical spine) Lateral and medial epicondylitis Neck pain[a] Unilateral back pain Other knee, calf and foot pains; conditon labelled as Morton's metatarsalgia	Fibromyalgia Post-laminectomy syndromes Shoulder pain	Disease process, in inflammatory arthropathies including ankylosing spondylitis
Other painful conditions		
Tension-type headache Atypical facial pain Dental pain, with no obvious treatable dental cause Non-cardiac chest pain Trochanteric bursitis, condition labelled as meralgia paraesthetica	Chronic widespread non-specific back pain[a] Painful diabetic neuropathy, other painful peripheral neuropathies	Tinnitus Motor spasm after stroke Epilepsy Multiple sclerosis symptoms Parkinson's
Neurological		
Migraine	Spinal pain related to nerve root entrapment or impingement Neuropathic pain or pain from true neuromas Complex regional pain syndrome Ischaemic pain Phantom limb pain Raynaud's disease Neurogenic pain, e.g. trigeminal neuralgia Central ('thalamic') pain	
Abdominal conditions		
Dysmenorrhoea Irritable bowel syndrome presenting mainly as pain Irritative bladder syndrome	Symptoms of ulcerative colitis or Crohn's disease, irritable bowel syndrome presenting mainly as disturbance of bowel function Urinary incontinence	Bladder outlet obstruction Generalized or systemic skin conditions, e.g. psoriasis
Conditions without pain		
Nausea Hay fever, allergic rhinitis Xerostomia, dry eyes Menopausal hot flushes Reversible local skin conditions		

[a]Symptoms and signs of neurological involvement make a response less likely.
This table is based on clinical experience, case series and randomized controlled trial evidence and, therefore, includes the possible benefits of the effects of the expectation associated with acupuncture.

If the expectations of both the patient and the practitioner are positive, then success seems more likely – though acupuncture can certainly be effective in patients who seem to have very low expectations of it helping. It is important for practitioners' expectations for acupuncture to be realistic and to make sure that patients who have unrealistic ones can be gently disabused without having their hopes completely dashed.

Acupuncture equipment

Standard needles

Acupuncture needles consist of a shaft and a handle. The shaft is generally stainless steel sometimes coated in silicone; and handles may be of metals or plastic, as shown in Plate 1. The various features of the needles are listed in Table 11.2.

There have been reports that silicone fragments may break off the surface coating and (theoretically) provoke foreign body reactions, but this is a risk common to all silicone-coated hypodermic needles and surgical instruments, not just acupuncture needles.

The needle tip does not simply taper to a point like a pencil, but has a rounded profile (traditionally likened to a pine cone) shown in Figure 11.1. This is supposed to be less traumatic – pushing tissue fibres apart rather cutting them – but it can still damage blood vessels, nerves and other structures if the needle or the patient moves. The modern needle is manufactured to a high standard, but occasionally the point is blunt or hooked, or the handle not firmly attached to the shaft. Such needles should be rejected as soon as the problem is discovered.

The typical diameter and length (which refers to the exposed part of the shaft, not including the handle) of acupuncture needles commonly used are shown in Table 11.3.

Only purchase single-use disposable needles.

TABLE 11.2

Variations in needle manufacture

Part	Variations	Advantages/disadvantages
Shaft (stainless steel)	Unpolished	Standard: 'gripped' by the tissues to produce *de qi*
	Polished Silicon-coated	Patient comfort, but less grip on tissues so *de qi* may be more difficult to elicit
Handle	Wound metal (steel, copper)	Easy to manipulate
	Solid metal	Less easy to manipulate
	Plastic	Lightweight[a] but non-conductive

[a]In some positions, a needle that is lying superficially will be more likely to fall out if the handle is heavy steel, in which case lightweight plastic can be an advantage.

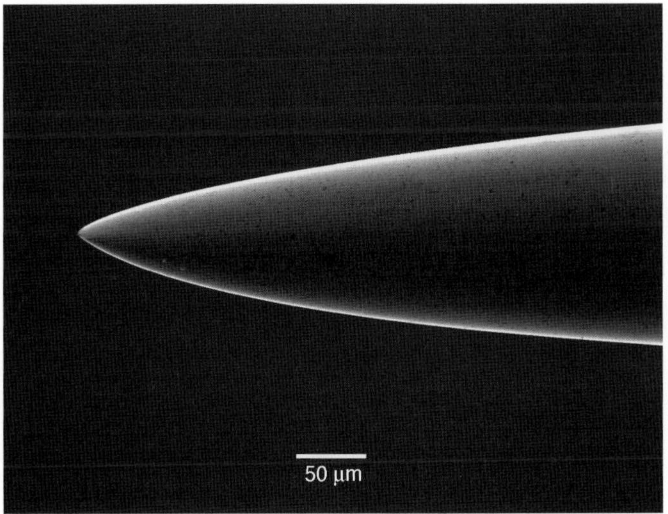

Figure 11.1 Electronmicrograph of acupuncture needle tip (courtesy of Plymouth University).

TABLE 11.3

Variations in dimensions of needles commonly available

	Range	Standard	Special purposes
Diameter	0.12–0.35 mm	0.25 or 0.30 mm	Longer needles should be thicker, for strength; typically 0.30 or 0.35 mm
Length	7–125 mm	25 or 40 mm	Longer lengths up to 75 mm are used for deep points, e.g. in the gluteal muscles Shorter lengths, 15 mm, are used in the face and ear

Guide tubes

Traditionally, needles were inserted directly using a deft flick-and-twist action, but now most needles are available with plastic guide tubes, and these are recommended for beginners. The needle is about 2 mm longer than the tube, enough to allow it to be inserted through the skin by tapping the end. Single needles are usually held in the guide tube with a wedge or plug. After freeing the needle, tip the guide tube so the handle appears, and hold it between finger and thumb to stop it falling out.

Other types of needle

Indwelling needles are sometimes used to continue the effect of treatment between attendances at clinic. There are special contraindications and precautions for using them, which we discuss in Chapter 13. The most common form of indwelling needle is like a tiny drawing pin with a 2 mm projection

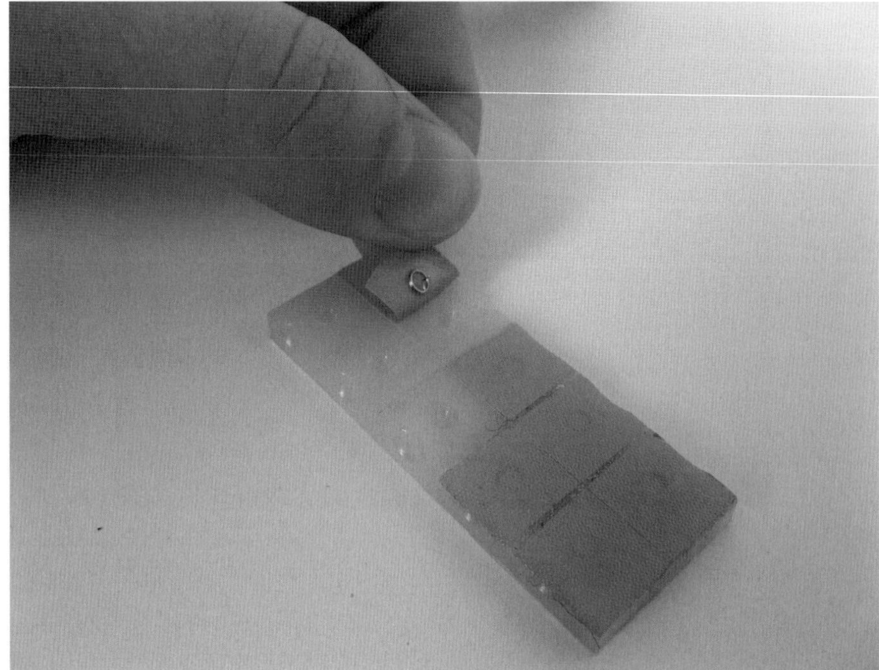

Figure 11.2 Photograph of indwelling needle with integral adhesive dressing.

(Plate 9). They are made in various diameters, and sometimes have an integral adhesive dressing (Fig. 11.2). They are sometimes used for auricular acupuncture (when they may be called 'press studs'), but we discuss the potential dangers of this below. They may also be used at other sites and need to be fixed securely with an adhesive dressing (Plate 10).

Auricular acupressure can be applied using stainless steel balls or, more traditionally, seeds of the *Vaccaria* plant, as shown in Plate 11.

Electroacupuncture equipment

While some practitioners never use electroacupuncture (EA) in the whole course of their professional career and, presumably, their patients are pleased with the results, most find that, before long, they want to be able to use EA particularly for patients with chronic pain.

Choosing EA equipment is not straightforward: cheap stimulators are available that are sometimes effective, but apparatus that is really flexible and reliable enough costs several hundred pounds. It is worth buying the best you can afford. Some of the most important criteria for a quality machine are suggested below (see Box 11.5). Some of the older models that are still available do not perform as described and might not meet current standard quality criteria; in Europe, standards are set by the International Electrotechnical Committee (CEI), but there are, as yet, no specific standards for EA machines. Modern apparatus is made to high standards (Plate 2) and have a maximum

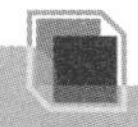

BOX 11.5

Suggested features of optimal electroacupuncture apparatus

- Low-voltage operation, preferably battery powered
- Master on/off switch
- Square wave output with waves of alternating polarity
- Low- and high-frequency outputs (e.g. 2–4 Hz and 80–100 Hz), with automatic switching between them
- Separate adjustment for the intensities of low-frequency and high-frequency outputs
- At least three pairs of output leads, each with its own intensity control
- Each intensity control placed in line with its output socket, for easy identification.

current of about 12 mA, which produces about one-tenth the maximum transthoracic electrical charge recommended by the US Food and Drug Administration (John Thompson, personal communication). Some employers insist that all new equipment should be checked by a hospital physics department or similar laboratory.

Ancillary equipment

It is essential to have the following close at hand when treating patients:

- Facilities to wash and dry the hands before treating each patient; alcohol gel is an acceptable alternative
- Couch and pillows to support the patient in the correct position
- Cotton wool swabs to press on the point after removing the needle
- Safe disposal boxes for used needles and swabs
- Facilities for keeping records.

Practitioners who use a separate side room for acupuncture, so they can leave patients relaxing during treatment, should have an intercom or call system for the patient, and a method of reminding themselves that there is a patient in the examination room.

Re-sterilizing needles

In certain circumstances where it is impossible to use single-use disposable acupuncture needles for one reason or another, the only way to deliver acupuncture may be to reuse needles after sterilizing them. Full, hospital-standard sterilization is absolutely essential in order to avoid transferring infection, e.g. hepatitis virus, between patients. Needles rapidly become blunt when repeatedly heated up during the sterilization process, and are then painful for patients.

The setting for acupuncture

Now that health clinics and hospitals in the West routinely meet high standards, it is easy to forget the relevance of the treatment setting to safe practice. In two cases reported in the literature, patients who were severely debilitated by chronic illness were given acupuncture at their own home in filthy conditions. They developed septicaemia, which ultimately contributed to their death.

The setting for acupuncture practice must offer the following facilities:

- For adequate examination: good light and good access
- For adequate treatment: anatomical landmarks must be identifiable, e.g. to establish the surface anatomy of the pleura; patient adequately supported on a firm surface so depth of insertion can be monitored (sometimes difficult in the patient's home, which constitutes a real hazard).

Other aspects of the setting that are relevant for safety include having adequate *time* to carefully conduct the procedure and having sufficient *active support* from other staff and colleagues.

Preparation of the practitioner

This is a checklist of items that practitioners should reflect on before starting treatment, to ensure that they:

- have the knowledge and skill – both in medicine and in acupuncture – to treat the patient safely and appropriately
- have formed (or been informed of) a diagnosis and treatment plan
- in collaboration with the patient, judge that the potential benefits of using acupuncture in this patient's circumstances outweigh the risks
- have considered the possible effects of acupuncture on any other condition present
- have checked that the setting and equipment are satisfactory
- know the anatomical relationships of all the points they plan to treat
- can cope with all likely adverse events that might arise
- have indemnity insurance in place.

Finally, practitioners should ensure their hepatitis B immunization is up to date, not only to protect themselves, but also to protect their patients. One small cluster of hepatitis B infections was attributed to spread from the practitioner who was himself antigen positive. This virus is highly infectious in minute doses.

Summary

This chapter is the first of three that are essential reading before using acupuncture in clinical practice: it describes and lists the conditions that must be present for you to make the decision to use acupuncture.

Acupuncture is contraindicated if the patient has a needle phobia or is not willing, and if the patient bruises spontaneously and has not had their clotting function checked. Particular acupuncture techniques are also contraindicated in certain situations: indwelling needles in patients with valvular heart disease, electroacupuncture when an intracardiac defibrillator is fitted. Relative contraindications require the practitioner and patient to balance the potential benefit and risk: severe bleeding tendency, significant psychological disturbance, compromised immune system, history of major seizure induced by a medical procedure and a marked previous reaction to acupuncture.

Special precautions need to be taken for particular patients such as those with bleeding disorders, epilepsy or immunosuppression. Pregnancy is not a contraindication, though certain techniques are best avoided. Patients without a clear diagnosis, or with any distorted anatomy, need careful consideration, as do patients who must drive after treatment. Strong reactors experience aggravation of their symptoms and other adverse effects after normal strength treatment and need to be treated lightly. It is difficult to predict reliably which patients will be strong reactors.

Patients must give their informed consent to treatment, which depends on being given adequate information tailored to their needs and abilities to understand. Consent is generally implied by the fact that patients make themselves ready for treatment, but signed consent may be required in particular circumstances.

Conditions that are suitable for acupuncture include many musculoskeletal conditions, particularly myofascial pain, but not systemic (inflammatory) arthritis. Also, soft-tissue injuries that are slow to heal may clear quickly with acupuncture. Some medical conditions may be mimicked by myofascial trigger point pain. Nociceptive pain generally responds better than neurogenic pain. Expectation may improve the outcome in painful and some non-painful conditions, but it is inappropriate to raise expectations excessively.

Non-painful conditions that may respond include nausea, allergies such as rhinitis, xerostomia and menopausal hot flushes.

Basic acupuncture equipment includes single-use disposable needles of various sizes. Vital ancillary equipment includes washing facilities, couch, cotton-wool swabs and sharps disposal box. Other specialized supplies may include electroacupuncture apparatus and auricular acupuncture needles.

The setting in which acupuncture is provided should be clean and conducive, permitting careful examination and treatment and providing necessary support and time.

Practitioners who give acupuncture are responsible for developing appropriate skills, knowledge and attitudes for safe and effective practice.

CHAPTER

12 Effective needling techniques

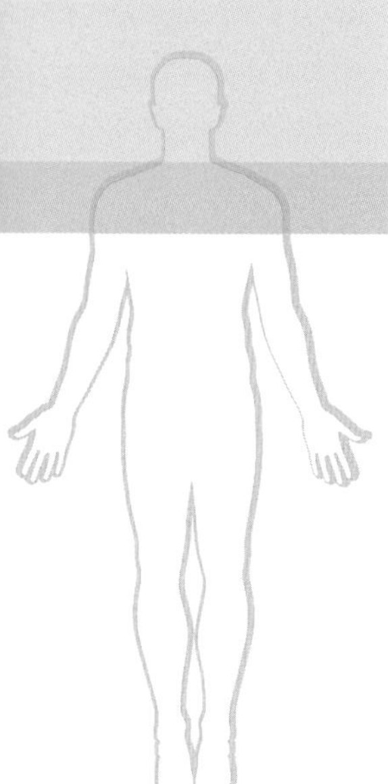

Contents

After reading this chapter you should be able to:

- perform standard manual needling of body points
- modify the dose of acupuncture for individual patient sensitivity
- manage a course of treatments.

Introduction

Do not start reading the book here! This chapter discusses the basic needling techniques for effective practice. It assumes that you have read Chapter 11, completed the preparatory checks, and understood the Western medical approach to acupuncture. Also, it is essential to read the following chapter on safety before starting practice, since safety is of equal importance to effectiveness.

Readers will be familiar by now with our suggestions for the 'standard' doses of treatment to activate the different mechanisms. This chapter describes a standard technique in more detail and the ways in which the dose can be adjusted for the individual patient. This adjustment has to be judged for each patient individually according to the responses – both the immediate response to the needle stimulation, and the effects that they experience over the next few hours and days, in both their symptoms and their general wellbeing. This chapter is about getting the dose of acupuncture right, though the best tutor is reflective clinical practice.

The methods of varying the dose of acupuncture (the strength of treatment) are mainly based on clinical experience rather than systematic research. As readers will expect, we do not consider all the finer variations in treatment that are described in books of traditional Chinese medicine, but cover what we believe to be reasonable according to current understanding. You will not, for example, find details about whether to rotate the needle clockwise or anticlockwise, but you will find a discussion of the strength of stimulation.

Dose of acupuncture

Effective treatment with acupuncture means choosing the point or points for this condition in this patient, and then needling them with a dose that achieves the right response without causing an adverse reaction. Our general recommendation is to start with a standard treatment in case the patient is sensitive, even if you anticipate that more needles with greater stimulation and longer retention will be needed: it is better to gradually increase the dose, once you know how the patient reacts. The treatment variables are shown in Table 12.1.

Practitioners must be clear on the simple ways to reduce the dose of treatment:

- Use thinner needles
- Use fewer needles
- Insert the needles superficially
- Reduce the amount of needle stimulation
- Reduce the time the needle is retained.

Acupuncture: basic technique

Standard manual acupuncture, i.e. the insertion of a needle into the tissues usually with some form of stimulation, is the most commonly used form of acupuncture throughout the world. The aim is to produce an adequate stimulation in the safest and least painful way. We describe the process in five phases:

1. Insert the needle through skin
2. Advance the needle to the required depth, usually in a perpendicular direction
3. Manipulate the needle, if required
4. Retain the needle in situ, if required
5. Remove the needle.

No needle should be inserted without preparation (Chapter 11) and without considering safety (Chapter 13) including, for example, the posture of the patient and the practitioner's anatomical knowledge.

TABLE 12.1

Factors involved in the strength of sensory stimulation that may affect the dose of an acupuncture treatment

Treatment variable	Range
Type of point	Myofascial trigger points (MTrPs) are 'strongly effective' when very active (painful), and relevant to the presenting complaint For other points, the major classical points such as LI4 are strongest, followed by classical points, and local non-traditional points are weakest
Number of points	Minimum treatment involves one point only; usual treatment involves between 4 and 10 points
Needle type	Larger diameter may have greater effect; highly polished surface reduces effect
Number of needle insertions	Each insertion counts separately
Depth of insertion	Increasing strength from superficial to muscular and further to periosteal levels
Needle stimulation	Increasing from none, to manual once, manual several times, and finally to electrical stimulation
Responses elicited	Amount of *de qi*, twitch response of muscle, or muscle contraction with electroacupuncture
Needle retention time	Longer is generally considered to be stronger, up to about 30 minutes maximum
Treatment frequency	Usually weekly, or twice weekly, but may be up to 5× per week
Total number of treatments	Typical courses are about six sessions, but sometimes long-term intermittent 'top-up' treatments are necessary to maintain relief

Insertion

This should be swift and painless; use the guide tube supplied with needles and tap the needle handle with confidence (Fig. 12.1). Tell patients that they will feel the tap but they probably will not notice anything sharp – though they may do occasionally, particularly if the skin is hot and sweaty. If there is a sharp pain, then the needle has hit a nerve, or a richly innervated vessel wall, or fascial layer. Try adjusting the needle first, either a little deeper or move superficial, but if the pain does not settle then remove it. If the pain continues even after removing the needle, one of the best ways to stop it is to swiftly reinsert the needle close to the site. This usually stops the pain, but you need to be confident in your actions.

Establish the habit of counting the number of needles inserted (*and* their guide tubes), preferably twice, and recording the number in an orderly way so you can check later that you have taken all the needles out – again counting twice to help avoid human error.

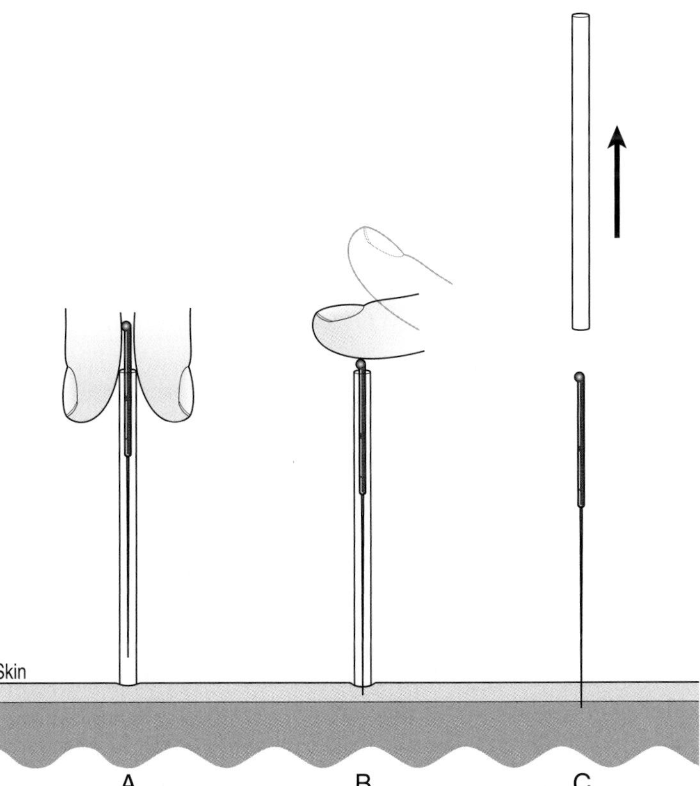

Figure 12.1 Diagram indicating that the needle can be held securely in the guide tube if it is slightly retracted, and that a smart tap with the finger tip will insert the needle subcutaneously, allowing the guide tube to be carefully lifted away.

Advance

Once inserted, the needle is situated in the subcutaneous tissue; it will hang sideways if not supported, and it can be left there for 'superficial' needling. But it needs to penetrate deeper either to elicit *de qi* or to inactivate a trigger point. Most acupuncture points are situated over muscle, and a few over loose connective tissue (for example BL60 and KI3, just anterior to the Achilles tendon). Usually, therefore, the needle is advanced into the muscle layer; and slight resistance can be felt as it passes through the fascia.

The direction of advancement is usually perpendicular to the skin: important exceptions are when needling over the rib cage and sternum (see below).

Manipulation

The needle can be manipulated with two techniques, illustrated in Figure 3.3:

1. 'Lift and thrust', i.e. repeated vertical movements of about 1–2 cm. (This is also known as 'sparrow pecking'.)
2. Rotation – rapid rotation about 90° in alternate directions using index finger and thumb.

Do this until the patient feels *de qi*. Often, at about the same time, the tissues grip the needle. The components of *de qi* are described in Chapter 2: most practitioners do not tell patients exactly what to expect so as not to bias their description of the sensations.

The individual needling response is quite variable, though we do not understand why, and there are some patients in whom it is difficult or impossible to achieve *de qi* at all. If you cannot elicit *de qi* in a patient for whom you think it is necessary, reinsert the needle a few millimetres away and try again. More than two or possibly three insertions at one location are enough for any patient.

The technique for inactivating MTrPs is slightly different and is described below.

If any manipulation becomes unpleasantly painful or aversive, stop.

Please note that some practitioners choose not to manipulate the needles at all, once they have been inserted to their desired depths (including one of the editors!)

Retention

There is a long tradition in acupuncture treatment of leaving patients lying quietly with their needles in situ for about 20 minutes ('needle retention'), which tallies with the time taken for CSF β-endorphin concentrations to reach their maximum levels. Needles are usually left for this time for segmental, extrasegmental and central effects. However, good responses may be obtained after 10 minutes. Treatment of MTrPs does not need to be prolonged, and clinically many cases with tender points other than trigger points seem to respond to a few minutes' needling, perhaps through the axon reflex (see Chapter 3). Patients can relax deeply in about 10 minutes, but 20–30 minutes lying down is even more likely to result in relaxation or sedation if you have the facilities to allow this.

Removal

Usually each needle can be pulled straight out; many practitioners then press briefly on the point with a cotton wool ball (not a finger – you could spread infection, such as hepatitis), to stem any tiny spot of bleeding. Sometimes needles become bent by muscle contraction, which may be due to electroacupuncture (EA) or the patient's own movement. Bent needles have to be coaxed out more carefully. Very occasionally a needle breaks accidentally, and if it could cause damage to particularly vital structures (e.g. pleura, spinal cord, eye) then it could constitute a surgical emergency. The needle must be removed in any event underimaging, unless the tip is visible to the naked eye when buried in soft tissue.

Finally, check that all the needles have been removed and safely placed in a sharps container.

Guide tubes should also be accounted for, since patients or cleaners may be unfamiliar with the apparatus and may regard them as dangerous.

Count the needles in, twice; count the needles out, twice.

Acupuncture: variations on the basic technique

Needling myofascial trigger points

If the myofascial trigger point (MTrP) is acutely tender and the pain is intense (signs of a highly active MTrP), then needle it cautiously.

In normal cases, fix the MTrP with one finger either side of, or along, the band and advance the needle onto the MTrP, keeping eyes and fingers ready to identify a twitch response. This has been shown to predict a good response, as does a reproduction of the patient's pain (Hong et al 1997). Often the MTrP will not be found first time, or several MTrPs will be present in one muscle: in both cases it will be necessary to re-advance the needle at a slightly different angle, exploring the muscle in a fan-like pattern (Fig. 12.2) – but avoid withdrawing it completely from the body, to save having to reinsert it through the skin. When no more twitches can be produced, withdraw the needle and press the area to prevent bleeding within the muscle, as this causes post-treatment soreness.

Choose a needle that is long enough to reach the MTrP: for example, piriformis cannot be reached with the standard 30 mm needle and needs one of at least 70 mm.

Superficial needling

In Japan, particularly for non-painful conditions, needles are usually inserted into the points subcutaneously, without stimulation. This technique is also used by many practitioners in the West, and called 'minimal' or 'superficial' acupuncture (Baldry 1993, Mann 1992). In Japan the needles are retained for 20 minutes or so, but in the West practitioners who use superficial

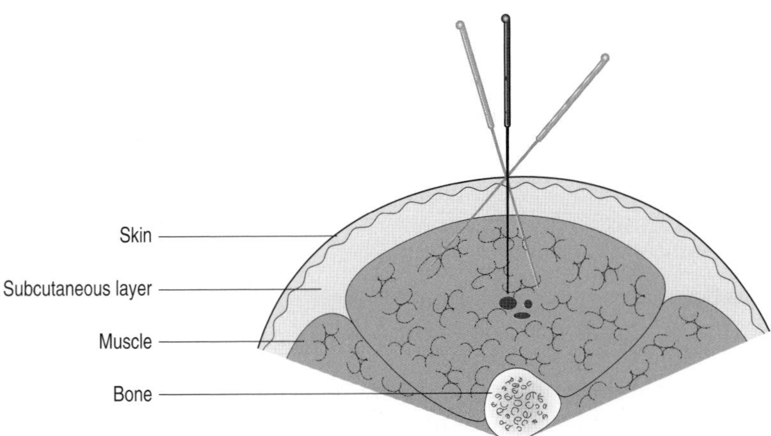

Figure 12.2 Diagram illustrating in principle how to explore fan-wise with a needle to eliminate all parts of a myofascial trigger point. The needle is withdrawn only as far as the subcutaneous layer, so that it does not need to be reinserted through the skin.

acupuncture generally state that as little as half a minute may be enough to produce treatment effects. Baldry describes this as a useful method of de-activating trigger points.

Periosteal pecking

In contrast to superficial needling, a strong treatment has evolved in the West. It is called 'periosteal pecking' and involves choosing a point where the bone is readily within reach of the needle (usually around joints, e.g. the tibial plateau distal to the anteromedial aspect of the knee joint line). The location should be chosen for its segmental effects, as shown in the Table 16.3. Then advance the needle tip until it touches the periosteum, and just tap the periosteum a few times before removing the needle. It is important to take care not to use more than a few touches, since periosteal pecking can produce strong reactions, especially in younger patients. We advise practitioners to gain skill in handling needles in different tissues before they attempt periosteal pecking.

Electroacupuncture

Origins

EA developed in its modern form in China in the 1950s, specifically for use in surgical operations. When acupuncture was first used for analgesia, the anaesthetists had to continue to rotate needles manually throughout the operation, so they developed EA apparatus to relieve themselves of this chore. Although EA analgesia was initially used quite widely in China and caused a great deal of interest in the West, subsequently a clearer picture of its true value has emerged: EA may help reduce the requirement for intraoperative and postoperative analgesic drugs, but does not on its own produce a response reliably. Some patients gain a considerable rise in pain threshold, others none at all.

The decision to use EA in practice is personal: some practitioners argue that EA goes against the spirit of a 'natural' therapy, and that they can achieve all the results they need with manual needling alone. Other acupuncturists find EA useful, particularly for patients with chronic nociceptive pain who have failed to respond to one or two sessions with manual needling, and for central stimulation (Fig. 12.3). Other possible roles for EA are as an adjunct to surgical analgesia, and in treatment of drug addiction.

Application

When intending to use EA, insert the needles in the usual way, but plan their placement so that pairs of needles can be connected together by pairs of leads from the apparatus. Most apparatus offers three or four pairs of leads that can be connected at the same time. It is not easy to give comprehensive advice on the practical aspects in a book, and courses on EA are available. For treating areas of pain, the needles can be connected across the site in order to 'flood'

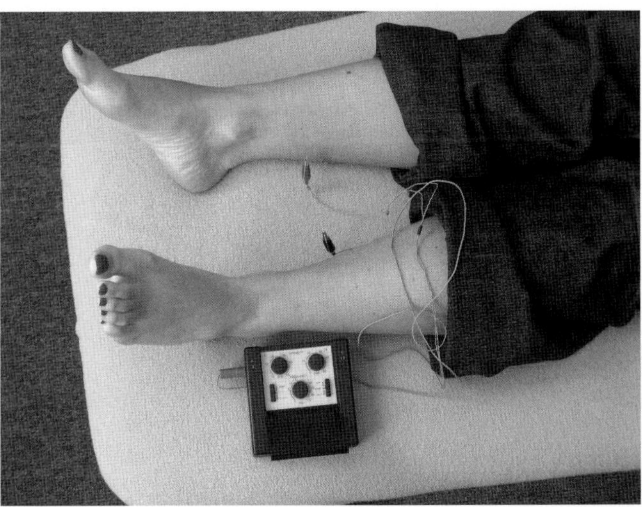

Figure 12.3 Electroacupuncture being given via a pair of leads attached to SP6 on each leg.

the area with current. When treating an MTrP, one lead attaches to the needle in the point, and its pair to a neutral needle at any other site.

A wise practitioner double checks that the apparatus is switched off before connecting the leads, then gradually increases the strength of treatment while checking what the patient feels. The two parameters that can be controlled are the frequency and the intensity:

- *Frequency*. This usually ranges from 2 to 80 or 100 Hz. The most common arrangement is 3-second periods alternating between 2–4 Hz and 80–100 Hz. This pattern is designed to prevent nerve accommodation, and to maximize the variety of neurotransmitters released.
- *Intensity* of the electric current. Increase the intensity from zero slowly, firstly until the patient is aware of it and then further until either it causes muscle twitch or it becomes as much as the patient can tolerate comfortably. When using two alternating frequencies, the patient may sense one frequency but not the other; this is where it is particularly useful if the apparatus allows separate intensity settings for each frequency.

Treatment is usually given for about 20–30 minutes. The response may tail off after the first few minutes, in which case the intensity must be increased again. Some patients may be willing and able to adjust the intensity for themselves. Occasionally, the intensity suddenly becomes strong – usually because the patient has moved, presumably bringing the needle closer to a nerve. Patients need to be informed about this possibility. Figure 12.4 shows EA being used to treat facet joint pain.

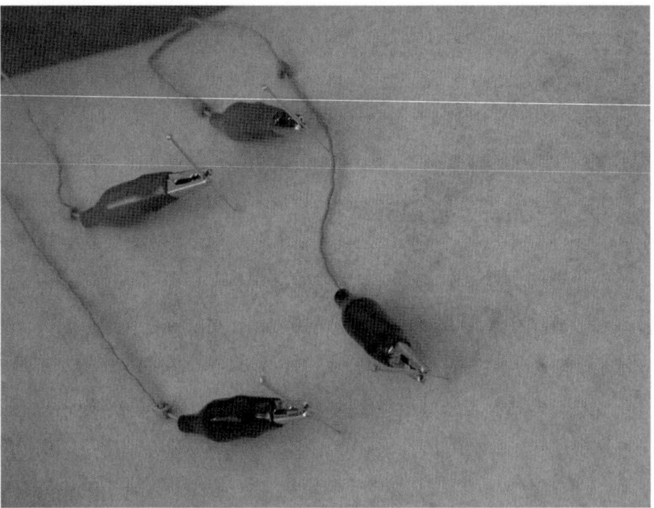

Figure 12.4 Electroacupuncture being used to treat facet joint pain.

Safety of electroacupuncture

EA should not be used if the patient is at all nervous about electrical stimulation. In the USA it is not allowed to connect needles across the head or neck. Do not use EA in areas of sensory denervation.

It is questionable whether EA can affect the function of the conducting system of the heart, or artificial pacemakers. A case was reported in which an ECG tracing was interpreted as showing that a cardiac pacemaker was affected by EA (Fujiwara et al 1980), but this may not be the correct interpretation. Calculations show that EA only generates an electrical charge around the heart of one-tenth the maximum recommended by the FDA. But the factors that control the intensity of the electrical field – type of current, skin thickness, needle type and depth of insertion – are still not known, so it is sensible to be cautious. We firmly recommend not connecting needles electrically across the thorax (either the chest wall or from arm to arm).

EA should also be used cautiously in patients with epilepsy. EA in the region of the carotid sinus or the vagus nerve in the anterior triangle of the neck may cause bradycardia; and EA near the recurrent laryngeal nerve may cause laryngeal spasm. EA to the scalp has been reported to cause angina pectoris. The symptoms recurred when the treatment was repeated, but no mechanism has been offered to explain this observation.

Individual patient sensitivity

Patients vary in their response to acupuncture, and some readily experience feelings of fatigue or malaise or a worsening of symptoms, as we discussed in the section on strong reactors in Chapter 11.

There is no definite way to anticipate who will react strongly, so the most sensible approach is a therapeutic trial with all patients: do not overstimulate on first treatment and then, if there has been no reaction, increase the strength of subsequent treatments. As a general guideline, it would usually be safe to start with no more than four or five needles, stimulated once, and not left longer than 10 minutes.

A few patients will have a severe reaction even to this cautious treatment and then it is sensible to discuss with them the therapeutic options: either to give a lighter treatment next time (down to the bare minimum treatment with one small diameter needle retained for only 30 seconds) or to abandon treatment.

Managing the course of treatment

Acupuncture is often given as a course during which its effects accumulate. However, relatively acute musculoskeletal conditions, including MTrPs and other soft-tissue injuries that have failed to heal after (say) 6 weeks, may respond after just one or two treatments.

Second and subsequent treatments are guided by the response to earlier treatments. Most frequently, your patient will have noted some benefit, but it probably did not last. Repeat the treatment with slightly increased dose to achieve cumulative benefit for more profound and longer-lasting effects.

For most conditions, patients and practitioners should be prepared to commit themselves to a course of about six to eight treatments – fewer if symptoms are of recent onset and limited to one area, but more for chronic or extensive conditions. When pathology such as arthritis is present, treatment will probably have to be continued with 'top ups' at increasing intervals, initially monthly, but then less frequently.

Not all patients respond to acupuncture, of course. If there is no response to the first session, check the history and examination, then increase the strength of treatment. If there is still no response, it is worth modifying the treatment approach appropriately – adding extrasegmental or central points, for example, or adding EA. If there is no sign of response within the first four sessions, most practitioners will abandon acupuncture; though some argue that a few patients may not start to respond until they have had six sessions.

If you are treating a patient with cancer who suddenly starts not responding to treatment that previously was effective, then consider the possibility that this is a sign of increasing tumour burden or recurrence.

Summary

This chapter describes the basic acupuncture technique and how to modify this technique to increase or decrease the dose of treatment, as required for each individual patient. The aim is to give sufficient dose to achieve a response, but not so strong that it produces a reaction. The dose can be tailored to the individual clinical circumstances in a number of ways, including the type and number of acupuncture point, needle type and number, depth of insertion, amount of stimulation, and the duration of treatment.

Once the patient has been correctly positioned, the basic manual technique consists of: insertion, advance, manipulation, retention and removal. The unique needle sensation known as *de qi* should usually be elicited. Needles should be counted in and counted out.

The standard needling technique can be modified for inactivating myofascial trigger points, for superficial (minimal) needling and for periosteal pecking.

Electroacupuncture (EA) is mainly used for central stimulation and to treat chronic pain and other conditions. The apparatus is attached to needles in pairs and the frequency and intensity of stimulation adjusted. Precautions for use of EA include not running current across the chest, not interfering with cardiac pacemaker or defibrillator, and (in the USA) not applying stimulation to the head.

Patients vary in their sensitivity to needling, and it is not easy to predict who will experience a reaction.

Treatment usually needs repeating up to about six to eight times to produce a cumulative and lasting effect. If there has been no response, a stronger treatment should be used and then other approaches should be tried. Most practitioners stop treatment if there has been no response whatsoever after four sessions, though a small minority of patients only start to show a response after six sessions.

CHAPTER

13

Safe needling

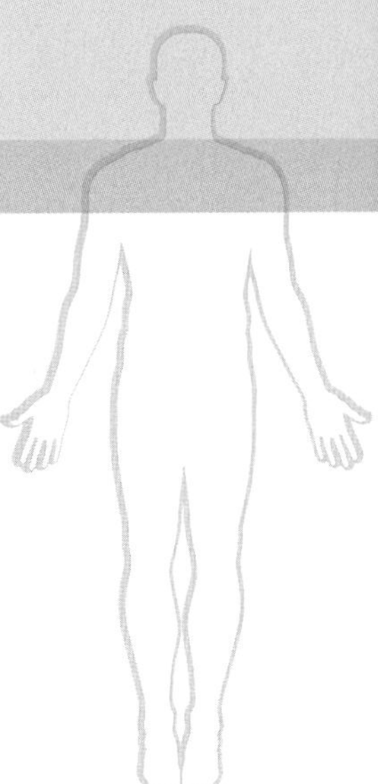

Contents

After reading this chapter you should be able to:

- state how to avoid injury to blood vessels, heart, peripheral nerves, spinal cord, pleura and lungs, and the abdominal organs
- state which particular patients are at risk of infection
- state which sites are particularly prone to infection.

Introduction

It is hardly necessary to emphasize the importance of safety, which should become integral to the practice of acupuncture. This chapter should be read in conjunction with the lists of overall contraindications and precautions in Chapter 11, Preparation for treatment. Advice is given on particular rules and techniques that are designed to avoid the most common adverse events that are reported in the literature.

Treat patients lying down

The final preparation before needling patients is to position them correctly. Ideally, they should be lying down at least for the first treatment, to avoid fainting. Fainting can cause serious consequences (including seizure), interrupts treatment and upsets patients. Occasionally, it may be impossible to gain access to the points that are needed, for example the neck and shoulders, when the patient is supine. In these cases patients may be treated cautiously sitting on the couch so that they can be laid flat immediately if they feel faint.

Check the face for pallor or sweating and the pulse for bradycardia. If you need to lie the patient down, remove all needles instantly.

Treat patients lying down, at least the first time.

Equipment and administration

Handling needles

In most cases, needles are used once and then disposed of in the sharps bin. In the case of brief needling (for example, treating MTrPs), then you may re-insert a needle, although beware that it rapidly becomes blunt and more painful when it crosses the skin and fascial layers. If a guide tube is used, the needle must be resheathed handle first – not sharp end first – to avoid needle-stick injury (Fig. 13.1).

As a general principle, a needle should either be in its original packet (unopened), in your hand in the guide tube, with the sharp end facing the patient, in a suitable point in the patient (during treatment), or in the sharps box. No needle should be left out of its packet lying unattended on any surface. Do not keep a patient's needles between treatment sessions, because the small saving in cost does not justify the risk of cross-infection associated with errors of handling. Guide tubes should not be shared between patients, again because of the small risk of cross-infection, so dispose of them after each patient contact.

Forgotten patients

Another event that is embarrassingly common is forgetting a patient who is being treated in a side-room. It is easy to see how this can occur: a doctor, for example, in primary care is running a busy surgery and puts a patient in

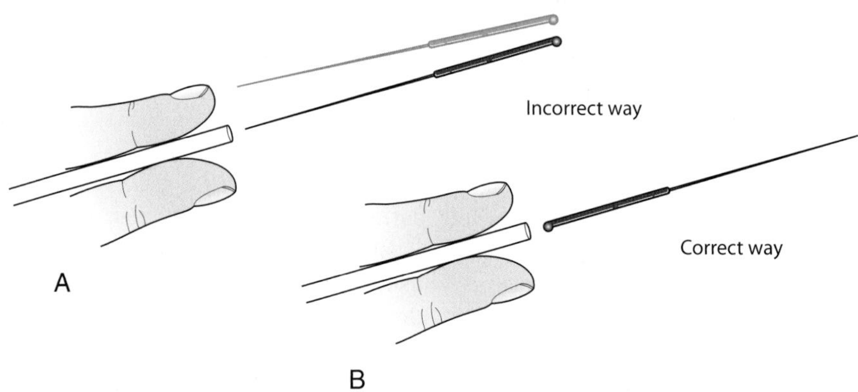

Figure 13.1 Diagram showing the risk of needle-stick injury on resheathing a needle: always resheathe handle first.

the side-room to allow more time for the acupuncture treatment. The doctor is called away on an urgent visit, and the patient is forgotten.

If the patient is treated in a side-room, install a system so that the patient can call for help. It is also wise to set up a reminder system in the main surgery to indicate that the side-room is occupied by a patient with needles.

Reducing the risk of trauma

The following sections are organized according to the structure at risk. This chapter does not claim to be totally comprehensive; for example, it does not address all the risks associated with all acupuncture points, only those that are likely to be used by the beginner. It does assume some knowledge of anatomy and readers are also recommended to study carefully three articles that discuss details of human anatomy specifically for the acupuncturist (Peuker & Cummings 2003a, 2003b, 2003c). Ultimately, the responsibility for safe practice rests with the practitioner.

Blood vessels

In the skin, reduce the risk of bleeding by avoiding needling into visible veins, and by paying attention to swift, clean insertion and removal. Stop any bleeding quickly in the normal way by pressing with a clean swab or tissue and elevating the part, as appropriate. Haematomata can be uncomfortable and unsightly, especially in the neck and face. Have a swab ready to press any speck of blood after removing the needle. You should press on a bleeding spot for up to 2 minutes to reduce the likelihood of a bruise.

It is important to avoid needling larger blood vessels, particularly at the elbow and popliteal fossa. This is not just because of the risk of bleeding: in fact, serious bleeding is rare since the needle makes a clean hole, provided the limb has not moved too much while the needles were in position (e.g. electroacupuncture can make the part twitch), and bleeding is usually easily staunched by pressure. However, arterial damage from needles has occasionally been reported to cause traumatic aneurysms: acupuncture to BL54/40 in the popliteal fossa caused an aneurysm of the popliteal artery that resulted in persistent symptoms of intermittent claudication. Similarly, a retroperitoneal haematoma has been reported as a result of bleeding from renal artery aneurysms that were produced by deep lumbar needling for back pain, and in another case the aorta was needled directly.

Before needling near a superficial artery, always identify the position of the artery by feeling for the pulse.

Deep vein thrombosis has also been reported at the site where a patient had been treated with acupuncture. Clearly this is difficult to prevent, although the less mobile patients should be encouraged to move actively after treatment.

The vertebral artery is vulnerable to needling of GB20 (for point locations, see Chap 16) and possibly BL10 in patients with slim necks, in whom the distance from the skin is less than the usual 4–6 cm; at GB20, a needle should not be inserted deeper than 3 cm in these patients, and should be angled upwards towards the base of the occiput – and towards the contralateral eye.

Heart

The blood vessels on the surface of the heart are within the reach of a standard acupuncture needle: if these vessels are penetrated, they may bleed into the pericardial space where pressure rapidly builds up – a condition known as cardiac tamponade, which is likely to be fatal. There are two reported deaths from tamponade after acupuncture. Practitioners must be very clear that they know where their needles risk touching the heart:

- Between the ribs over the anterior chest
- Sternal foramen (congenital abnormality).

Some 5–8% of the population have a congenital abnormality, the *foramen sternale*, which occurs when the two sides of the sternum fail to join together completely during ossification (see Plate 12). Usually this occurs at the fourth intercostal space, where the acupuncture point CV17 is located. When a foramen is present, the heart is only about 15–25 mm below the skin surface in slim patients, well within reach of the standard acupuncture needle (measurements from Elmar Peuker). The distance from the skin to the posterior surface of the sternum in one slim woman who died of cardiac tamponade was measured at post-mortem, and was between 13 and 19 mm. A foramen abnormality does not show on normal chest X-ray films, only on CT, and cannot reliably be detected by palpation. Therefore, CV17 must always be needled either superficially or obliquely at a maximum angle of 30° to the sternum.

Although tamponade has been reported from a needle between the ribs, practitioners should not in any case be needling between the ribs on account of the much more common risk of pneumothorax.

Peripheral nerves

Very occasionally, needling produces local symptoms – usually numbness or motor weakness, occasionally pain – that may persist for several weeks, presumably from neuropraxia. It is not clear why this happens in some cases, and it seems unavoidable. It may be commonest at LI4.

One place where needle injury can affect nerve function is the common fibular nerve, close to GB34, where it can cause foot-drop. Sometimes the sciatic nerve is needled directly when treating the piriformis muscle, or GB30 or BL54, causing sharp shooting pain, though rarely any loss of function. The median nerve is easily reached by a deep needle at PC6. In all such cases, the needle should be withdrawn from the nerve immediately, and the patient reassured. It seems likely that acupuncture needles impale nerves fairly frequently, but only rarely do any harm.

Spinal cord and brainstem

The spinal cord and roots of the spinal nerves are vulnerable to deep needling at the paravertebral Bladder and *Huatuojiaji* points, which should be needled in a mediocaudal direction. In individuals of normal physique, the spinal cord is about 25–45 mm deep from the surface in the thoracic region and about 55 deep in the low lumbar spine and cauda equina. In the midline (GV points), a needle angled in a cranial direction can pass between the overlapping spinous processes, so needles should be directed caudally. Lesions to the spinal cord have occasionally been reported in Eastern literature. These injuries produce focal neurological signs or paraplegia.

Immediately below the occiput, the brainstem and the cerebellum are vulnerable to injury during needling. Even though there may be a tradition of deep needling in this area, we strongly advise not to needle deeply, and to direct the needle upwards (cranially, towards the base of the occiput) when needling in the midline (GV points). At GB20, needle upwards and medially, towards the opposite eye.

Pleurae

Pneumothorax is the most common serious or potentially serious event reported in association with acupuncture. The chest wall is about 20–40 mm thick in healthy people, but compression of soft tissues is likely to occur during needling, so a depth of 10–15 mm should be regarded as the maximum in places where there is no rib or scapula to protect the pleura. Pneumothorax is a particular risk for patients with cachexia or a thin chest wall, which is likely in anyone seeking treatment with acupuncture for chronic respiratory disease: in these cases no needle should go further than immediately subcutaneously.

A pneumothorax can be produced by needling anywhere within the surface anatomy of the lung, but particularly in the supraclavicular fossa and between the ribs.

When needling over the ribs, the risk must be reduced in one of three ways (Fig. 13.2):

1. Fix the skin (and trigger or acupuncture point) between the fingers with the fingers placed in the intercostal space either side of the rib; needle directly over the rib
2. Use only superficial needling
3. Insert the needle obliquely, at a tangent to the ribcage.

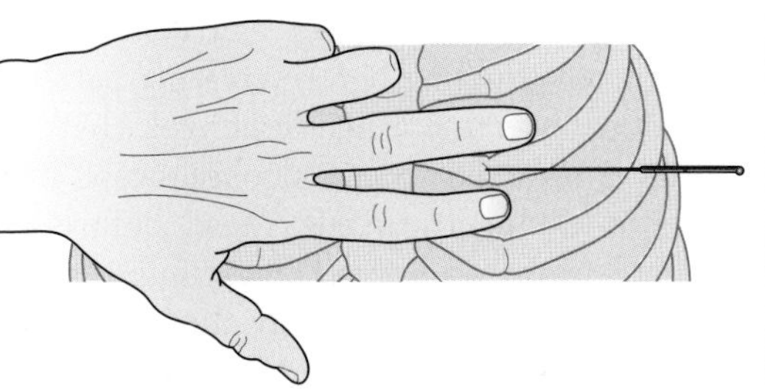

Figure 13.2 Diagram showing the technique for safe needling over the ribs: the trigger point has been fixed between the fingers, which are positioned over the intercostal spaces.

The point GB21 is frequently needled, and needs a particular technique, which is illustrated in Chapter 13.

Another point to note in relation to pneumothorax is the difficulty making the diagnosis: pneumothorax may only present some time, up to 2 days, after the injury. Anyone with pain, cough or shortness of breath within 2 days of acupuncture should be suspected of having a pneumothorax. X-ray examination should be arranged urgently to make the diagnosis and guide the management. Tension pneumothorax has occasionally been described after acupuncture and in this case emergency hospital treatment will definitely be needed. Although we describe these serious cases, it seems possible that a number of minor cases of pneumothorax occur after acupuncture without being identified and resolve spontaneously.

Abdominal organs

It is rare to see a report of penetration of the abdominal organs, though a recent case was described of deep needling in the epigastric region causing an aortoduodenal fistula, which resulted in the patient's death. As a guide to the safe depth of needle insertion, the abdominal wall is approximately 20–40 mm thick in adults of normal weight. It becomes thinner when stretched and thinner still when compressed during needle insertion.

Reducing the risk of infection

There are two main possibilities of how patients could become infected through acupuncture: contamination by bacteria from the skin of the patient or the practitioner, and transfer of blood-borne virus infection via needles contaminated with blood. Spreading infection between patients is eliminated by using single-use disposable needles.

Hygiene and skin preparation

Practitioners should always clean their hands with soap or alcohol gel before treating a patient with acupuncture and between patients. This is reassuring to patients and reduces the very occasional risk that the hands may be contaminated with methicillin-resistant *Staphylococcus aureus* or hepatitis B virus from a previous patient. Alcohol gel is only an effective substitute for soap if the hands are not visibly soiled, as alcohol does not penetrate organic matter. Practitioners should cover any wounds or skin lesions they may have with waterproof dressing before treating patients.

Before inserting a needle, check that the patient's skin is clinically clean. There is no need to use alcohol swabs routinely before acupuncture, just as there is no need to use them before giving injections (Hoffman 2001). Alcohol swabs do not reliably eliminate the bacteria on the skin surface, and have little effect at all on the bacteria deep within the glands, follicles and crypts of the skin. Anyway, skin flora is generally commensal and of low pathogenicity. Alcohol sensitizes the skin and makes needle insertion more painful. Long experience of injections without using swabs has shown no greater risk of infection. The number of bacteria that are likely to be inoculated on the tip of an acupuncture needle has been calculated to be well below that required to cause an infection in healthy patients (Hoffman 2001). This probably explains why infection after acupuncture is much less common than might be expected.

However, occasional cases of infection have occurred, ranging from cellulitis to necrotizing fasciitis. Infection is more likely in certain sites, and in debilitated or immunocompromised patients.

Long needles present a particular problem because the shaft needs to be supported while the needle is being advanced. Hold the shaft with a sterile swab, or support it by using a shorter guide tube (a new one, not one used for another patient).

The consulting room should be kept in a high standard of cleanliness; for example, blood spillages should be cleaned promptly. All non-sharp contaminated items should be discarded in a clinical waste bag (usually a yellow bag).

Vulnerable sites and vulnerable patients

Pay great attention in particular *sites* and in particular *patients*. The *sites* that are particularly vulnerable to infection include:

- cartilage of the ear (use a perpendicular insertion to avoid excessive damage to the cartilage)
- medial lower aspect of the leg, where varicose ulcers develop
- a limb with (or prone to) lymphoedema after cancer – avoid needling this limb
- a lower limb which has more than a trace of dependent oedema
- any area where the blood supply is compromised, for example by peripheral arterial disease
- other sites where an infection would be particularly devastating, such as joint spaces (including joint effusions, when present), fracture sites and the meninges
- where there is a foreign body such as a prosthetic joint.

The *patients* who are particularly at risk of infection include:

- immunocompromised patients, whether from conditions such as AIDS or as a result of immunosuppression therapy or cancer therapy
- those physically debilitated, e.g. from chronic illness.

One report has suggested that a patient with diabetes mellitus was at an increased risk of infections from acupuncture, but this seems likely to be an isolated case. Apart from increased vigilance no special action is necessary in patients with diabetes.

However, serious infections have very occasionally been reported in previously healthy patients with no apparent risk factors: we have to put this down to misfortune. Most opportunistic infections with acupuncture are caused by the *Staphylococcus* group. However, *Clostridia* species have been cultured from abscesses in the cervical spine and the temporomandibular region.

Bacterial endocarditis

Six cases of subacute bacterial endocarditis have been attributed to acupuncture. In five cases, the patients' heart valves were already abnormal following surgery or as a result of rheumatic fever. Three cases occurred after using indwelling needles, which are a recognized risk; but three occurred after sessions of normal body acupuncture, which is harder to explain (see above). The full circumstances of the acupuncture are unknown in these cases, as they were reported by staff unconnected with the treatment. No particular precautions are currently advised with regard to sessions of body acupuncture treatment in patients with heart valve abnormalities.

Indwelling needles are contraindicated in patients with valvular heart disease (including prosthetic valve) or past history of endocarditis.

Reducing blood-borne infection

There have been many cases in which hepatitis B virus has been transmitted from one patient to another by acupuncture needles that have been re-used without being properly sterilized. One report highlighted the poor sterilization procedures used in some practices (Walsh 2001). Epidemiological studies have shown a correlation between use of acupuncture and infection with hepatitis in some countries. We are not aware of case reports of infection with hepatitis C attributed to acupuncture, though there is the possibility that patients have been infected but remain asymptomatic (Walsh 2001).

Always use single-use disposable needles for acupuncture.

Similarly, there are four reports of spread of HIV with acupuncture needles, though these cases are all 'probable' rather than 'certain' (White 2004). Variant Creutzfeldt–Jakob disease is unlikely to be transmitted by acupuncture simply because the sites of infection (lymph nodes, tonsils, spleen and spinal cord) are not needled. However, the remote possibility of transmitting this disease, and the fact that the prion responsible is not killed by autoclaving, is another forceful argument against re-using needles.

Professional development

If something goes wrong, face up to it and discuss it frankly with the patient. Nobody gains if adverse events are concealed. Write a scientific report if it is serious or novel so that your colleagues can learn from it, and modify your practice procedures in the light of the experience. Keep any eye on the literature for new reports of adverse events associated with acupuncture so that you can incorporate any recommended changes into your practice.

Summary

Safety should be integral to the practice of acupuncture. Patients should normally be treated supine. Single-use disposable needles are obligatory. Patients who are left relaxing in a side-room are at risk of being forgotten, and ways of avoiding this must be arranged.

Trauma to organs should be avoided; blood vessels, heart, peripheral and central nervous tissue, pleurae and abdominal organs are particularly at risk.

Practitioners must take great care to prevent avoidable cases of infection, and wash their hands before treatment: the strictest aseptic technique is not necessary in normal cases. Particular care to avoid infection is recommended at the ear cartilage, in lymphoedema following surgery, gravitational oedema in the leg, anywhere the blood supply is compromised and near prostheses. Patients who are immunocompromised or debilitated are also at risk. Patients with heart damage are at risk of endocarditis with indwelling needles. Practitioners should be aware of the risk of transferring blood-borne infection and take steps to avoid this.

CHAPTER

14 Other acupuncture techniques

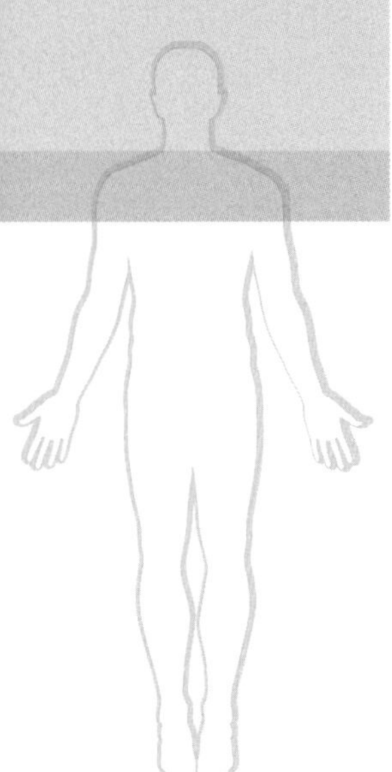

Contents

After reading this chapter you should be able to:

- describe how to use indwelling needles safely
- describe a rational approach to auricular acupuncture.

Introduction

Several different treatments have evolved under the heading of 'acupuncture and related techniques', including methods of continuous stimulation, different forms of stimulation, different models of treatment (microsystems) and electrical diagnostic methods.

The fact that a technique or piece of equipment is promoted and sold – or that it is included in this book – does not necessarily mean that it has been validated as an effective approach: most have not. Throughout the history of acupuncture, innovative practitioners have developed new ideas, probably for a variety of motives including personal prestige and business reward. It is necessary frequently to remind ourselves that a novel and unusual technique in the hands of a committed practitioner can have powerful expectation effects; we do not support the promotion of any novel technique as an effective treatment until it has been properly evaluated.

One of our purposes in including these techniques in this introductory book is to give a brief overview with a neutral, or even slightly sceptical, attitude, so that beginners are cautioned not to spend large sums on apparatus that offers to cure every ill, but then fails to live up to its promise.

However, there are two techniques that have some value: indwelling needles for continuous stimulation, and auricular acupuncture as a particular form of nerve stimulation.

Continuous stimulation by indwelling needles

One traditional technique in acupuncture, especially when treating patients with chronic pain, is to increase the strength of stimulation by inserting indwelling needles, which continue to stimulate the point between the treatment sessions. Nowadays, the most common type of indwelling needle looks like the outline of a drawing pin (US 'thumb-tack') as shown in Plate 9. These are also referred to as 'studs' especially when used in the ear. Various sizes are available, but the one with needle length of 2 mm is in most general use. Studs can be purchased with or without an adhesive dressing. Other methods are available for continuing the stimulation of the auricle, as we discuss below.

Of historical interest, the *umebari* technique from Japan was a rather notorious example of continuous stimulation: special, fine needles were inserted, then the handle portion was snipped off and the site massaged with the finger to drive the needle into the tissues. They were left there indefinitely. These *umebari* needles may be an incidental finding on X-ray examination many years later, or they can migrate around the body and cause trauma to distant tissues – kidneys and spinal cord have been reported. The Japanese professional acupuncture organizations effectively outlawed the procedure in 1976.

Safety of indwelling needles

There are three principal concerns about the safety of indwelling needles:

1. They may cause local infection, particularly of the ear.
2. They may cause bacteraemia, which may lead to endocarditis in susceptible patients (see Chapter 11).
3. If they fall out, there is a risk of transmitting blood-borne infection through needle-stick injury. Many patients are unaware that they are carriers of hepatitis B or hepatitis C virus, and so any indwelling needle that they lose constitutes a significant risk to public health that is impossible to manage.

Because of these concerns, the UK professional body (British Medical Acupuncture Society) does not recommend the use of indwelling needles unless they are used in a way that you can be sure is safe. Firstly, check that the patient does not have valvular heart disease or any other increased risk from bacteraemia (i.e. from severe debilitation or compromised immunity); secondly, make sure either that you know the patient is not a carrier of hepatitis B or C virus, or that the needles will not fall out. In practice, then:

- clean the skin thoroughly before inserting the needle
- cover the needle with a large and reliable dressing, e.g. a clear surgical dressing (Plate 10)
- instruct the patient fully on the reasons to make sure the needle is not lost.

Full details and instruction sheets are provided in a review paper (Filshie et al 2005). Devices, such as beads and seeds, that provide sustained acupressure rather than acupuncture are likely to be much safer (see below), but may be less effective.

Auricular acupuncture

Auricular acupuncture forms a special subsection of acupuncture; its theory and practice as well as the necessary precautions are sufficiently different from body acupuncture to justify its own section here, but there is only room to touch on part of the whole subject.

Background and concepts

A French acupuncturist, Dr Paul Nogier, discovered that local natural healers treated chronic back pain by cauterizing a particular area of the ear. Then, when one day the sun was shining across a patient's ear casting shadows, he noticed that the cartilage in that area consisted of a regular series of lumps that reminded him of the sacral spine. This gave him the idea that there might be some correlation between the ear and the rest of the body. He started examining the ears of all his patients, looking for a correlation between any spots, redness or tenderness in the ear and the patient's medical problem. He eventually derived the idea that the whole body is represented on the ear. This idea was soon adopted by the Chinese, acupuncturists throughout the world, and even the World Health Organization.

We are not convinced of the association, and are reminded of the fairy tale story of the Emperor's new suit. He ordered his tailor to make the perfect suit, but they found it impossible. Rather than admit it, they presented him with a set of invisible clothes, telling him that it was made of special cloth which was invisible to anyone who was stupid. The Emperor, so conscious of his image as to be devoid of common sense, believed them. His advisors also said they were convinced by the tailors' descriptions of the beautiful patterns and the intricate weave, since they were driven by the fear of being labelled as stupid if they could not see the clothes. The Emperor wore the (non-existent) clothes in public, and everyone collaborated in the charade, for fear of appearing stupid. It took the innocence of a small boy to announce: 'But he has nothing on at all'.

In charts of the original version, the body is represented upside down, like an inverted foetus; the head corresponds with the earlobe and the auricular canal with the umbilical cord. Nogier located the internal organs – the lung, heart, stomach, etc. – in the cavum concha, because it is usually innervated by the sensory branch of the vagus nerve. However, with further experience,

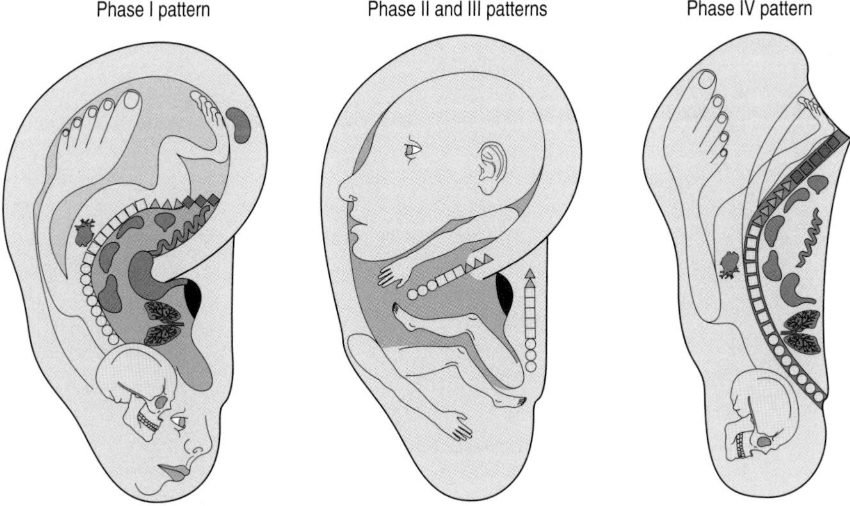

Figure 14.1 Different patterns of the supposed somatic representations on the ear, according to Nogier (from Auriculotherapy Manual by Terry Olson, reproduced with permission from the publishers Churchill Livingstone).

Nogier found that this pattern did not always explain his findings in patients, so he produced alternative charts – either with the body erect, or lying with the spine anteriorly – which could be used in patients whose ears did not match the first pattern; examples of these charts are shown in Figure 14.1, and readers can draw their own conclusions about the reliability of the method.

Western medical auricular acupuncture

Even though the idea of the body being represented on the ear has no physiological basis and attempts to validate somatotopic representation have not been convincing, that is not to say that acupuncture to the ear is of no value. Clinical experience suggests that stimulating the ear can produce useful clinical effects, even in cases that have not responded to standard, body acupuncture. The pinna is richly innervated by several nerves (shown in Fig. 14.2) and so is potentially a good site to stimulate the CNS in a direct, but rather general, way.

Treatment

There are several ways that practitioners of auricular acupuncture choose auricular points to needle: from the supposed correlations shown in published charts, or because they are tender, or because they show skin changes, particularly redness, or because they have a low electrical impedance. We cannot make firm recommendations about any of these.

Nogier used to insert the needle down to the cartilage and rotate it until the patient felt a burning sensation; this is not advisable because of the risk

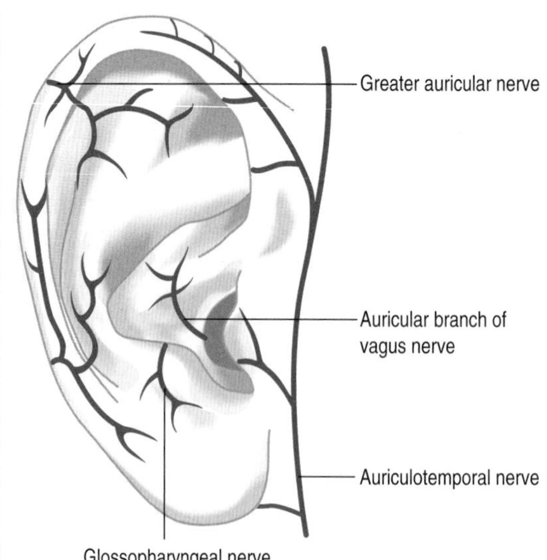

Figure 14.2 Diagram of the innervation of the auricle.

of injury to the cartilage and subsequent infection. Any stimulation with the needle should be gentle. Electrical stimulation can be used (though not in the USA, and not in patients with epilepsy), but the current should not be connected from one side of the head to the other.

Safe needling of the ear

Particular safety precautions for auricular acupuncture include the following:

- Take particular care to avoid infection in the ear, as once present it can be difficult to treat and may produce deformation of the cartilage.
- Insert needles perpendicular and superficially, to avoid damage to the cartilage.
- Do not use indwelling needles in any patient with valvular heart disease.

Approaches to continuous auricular stimulation

Indwelling needles or studs placed in the external ear have been used for treating either chronic pain or for smoking cessation, as discussed below. Another type of needle was developed specifically for the ear, which has a barbed end to help retain it in the skin; this seems unnecessarily traumatic, so we do not include an illustration. This needle is also magnetic, and is supposed to be stimulated by holding another magnet against it.

We do not recommend the use of any indwelling needle in the ear, because we have not yet found a reliable method of holding it in position.

Indwelling needles are difficult to retain in the ear reliably, which means they carry a high potential risk and blood-borne transmission. They also carry a high risk of local infection because they maintain a track for bacteria to migrate beneath the skin, and because the ear cartilage has a poor blood supply. For these reasons, pressure devices are sometimes used, such as *Vaccaria* seeds (Plate 11) and special small stainless steel balls, held in place by adhesive tape. In our experience, even these are not entirely free of the risk of local infection. Also, very occasionally they become deeply embedded and covered in a flap of skin, making removal difficult. Another problem is that auricular acupressure seems less effective than acupuncture.

NADA technique

One particular technique of auricular acupuncture is currently in widespread use in the USA and Europe for treatment of opioid and cocaine dependence. It evolved after an anaesthetist in Hong Kong, Prof. Wen, used electroacupuncture (EA) at auricular points for surgical analgesia in patients who happened to be addicted to opioids: he noticed that they hardly experienced any withdrawal symptoms in the postoperative period. Over time, the therapy spread to the USA and became what is known as the NADA (National Acupuncture Detoxification Association) technique. EA across the head was not favoured in the USA, so a manual technique was used. Conventional acupuncture needles are placed in five points in both ears (Fig. 14.3), while the patient sits in a chair in a quiet relaxing environment for up to 45 minutes, generally in a group with other addicts. Treatment is offered on a drop-in basis, and recovered addicts are trained to apply the treatment, keeping staff costs low.

The place of this treatment has always been clearly elucidated by Michael Smith, who was responsible for introducing it. He believes that the main

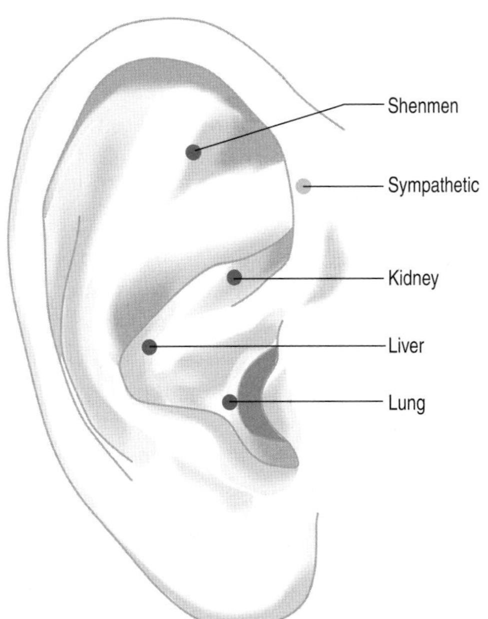

Figure 14.3 Points used in the NADA method of auricular acupuncture (Sympathetic point hidden in this view, on inner surface of helix).

value of auricular acupuncture in detoxification is to attract addicts with a therapy that helps them relax. In this way, they gain trust in the healthcare providers and are more likely to enrol in the various services that offer help in facing the problems associated with their dependency. Smith insisted that the NADA therapy on its own is not likely to be sufficient in achieving abstinence, and his view has been supported by the majority of the evidence from clinical trials.

Smoking cessation

Auricular acupuncture has also been widely adopted to help smokers quit smoking. The auricular points Lung and Shenmen (see Fig. 14.3) have been commonly used, and although evidence suggests that acupuncture at the correct site is no better than acupuncture at an incorrect site, acupuncture anywhere (in the ear) is clearly better than doing nothing to help the patient. The effect is not likely to be point specific.

Some studies have used indwelling needles (studs) or acupressure devices, as described above. The device is fitted on the quit-date, and the smokers are instructed to press the device with their finger whenever they feel cravings. There is some evidence to suggest that this stimulus may affect the release of dopamine in the nucleus accumbens, but whether that is the true mechanism of action, or whether acupuncture is simply a distraction, hardly matters if it helps achieve such an important target as stopping smoking.

Other stimulation techniques

Acupressure

Acupressure involves stimulating the body, usually at acupuncture points, with pressure from fingers, elbows or special devices. Various different approaches have originated in China, India, Korea and Japan, and they may have specific names, e.g. Shiatsu. Traditionally, hard wooden rods were used to apply real pressure! Some practitioners regard acupressure as a therapy in its own right, separate from acupuncture, though they often use traditional Chinese methods of diagnosis and treatment. The pressure used is quite considerable, and patients may feel bruised afterwards.

Sustained acupressure can be used for continuous stimulation, as a safer alternative to indwelling needles, discussed below. The traditional method involved taping seeds of *Vaccaria* to auricular points (see Plate 11). Presumably these seeds were chosen because they were an appropriate size.

More recently, after it was demonstrated that PC6 acupressure can reduce nausea particularly in pregnancy, special elasticated wristbands with a pressure dome have been available (Fig. 14.4). They are also promoted for seasickness, and similar wristbands are sold that stimulate HT7 with the aim of treating insomnia, though there has been no validation of this claim.

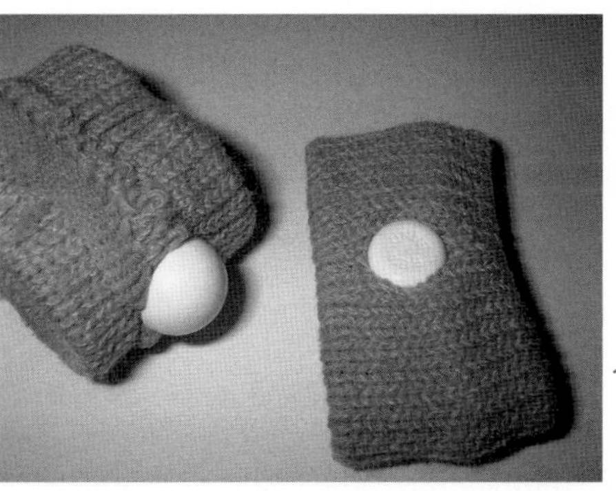

Figure 14.4 Photograph of commercially available wristband designed to apply pressure at PC6.

Moxibustion

Moxibustion is a traditional treatment used to warm either the needle or the skin itself (Plate 13). Moxa is a cotton-wool-like material made from the leaves of *Artemisia vulgaris,* which smoulders continuously rather than flaring up. It can be supplied:

- as loose 'punk', which is pressed round the needle handles or rolled into small *cones* burnt on the skin, either directly or on a slice of ginger
- rolled into a moxa *cigar,* the glowing end of which is held close to the acupuncture point, with or without the needle in situ.

We do not recommend the use of moxa: it constitutes a significant risk of burning the skin, and it makes an all-pervading, unpleasant smell. Traditionally in China, moxa was allowed to burn itself out on the skin, causing full-thickness blistering and permanent scar formation. Sometimes, more commonly in the USA, infra-red lamps are used to warm the needle, as a kind of modern version of moxa.

Plum-blossom needle

Plum-blossom needles consist of a number of short needles held close together with a long flexible plastic handle (Plate 14). This type of needle was used in the past to provide repeated stimulation to an area to produce erythema or bleeding, as a local treatment. The original plum-blossom needle was impossible to sterilize adequately, but disposable versions are now available.

Laser 'acupuncture'

Low-level lasers (i.e. lasers below the intensity that is needed to heat tissue) have been shown to have physiological effects, particularly in promoting the healing of skin ulcers. The light is directly absorbed by cells, but laser beams have not been shown to stimulate nerve endings. Acupuncturists became interested in lasers at the time of the initial AIDS scare in the 1980s, in the hope that they would offer an effective replacement for acupuncture needles. Another thing that made them popular at that time was significant reduction in their cost: lightweight and cheap crystals that produced light of a single wavelength became available, and soon replaced the original heavyweight laser generators.

Some early studies seemed to show that laser therapy could have systemic effects, and, somewhat uncritically, the idea developed that lasers could stimulate acupuncture points. There are theoretical doubts about this: the red laser, which was shown to have physiological effects, does not penetrate the skin more than a few millimetres, since it is absorbed by haemoglobin. The energy reaching the tissues may not be sufficient to adequately stimulate nerve endings. Infrared laser may penetrate further, but there is no clear evidence to show that this wavelength has beneficial physiological effects.

There is still considerable debate between practitioners on the optimal dosage (wavelength, power and duration) of laser therapy that should be used at acupuncture points. Nevertheless, there are persistent reports of double-blinded studies with positive results. The final verdict on whether laser may be effective in conditions such as headache and neck pain is still unknown. We suggest that practitioners should wait for more definitive evidence before using laser as a substitute for needles.

Transcutaneous electrical nerve stimulation

Transcutaneous electrical nerve stimulation (TENS) is sometimes included in descriptions of acupuncture. It consists of the application of electrical current to the body through carbonized rubber pads. The original frequency used was high, about 100 Hz or more, and only strong enough to produce a light tingling sensation. Later, the so-called 'acupuncture-like TENS' was developed using much lower frequencies (about 2 Hz) at strong enough intensity to cause muscle contraction.

In reality, even 'acupuncture-like TENS' is different from acupuncture as presented in this book. TENS was developed from theoretical considerations, i.e. knowledge that stimulation of Aβ fibres could inhibit pain transmission; acupuncture was developed by clinical tradition. TENS is used to treat pain, whereas acupuncture treats other symptoms too. TENS has an immediate effect, which is short term and has to be repeated, or used continuously; but acupuncture appears to have more lasting effects.

Gold and silver needles

Some manufacturers still provide needles made of gold or silver, which were supposed to 'stimulate' and 'drain' the patient's energy respectively. However, this interpretation is probably the result of a mistranslation from Chinese. Needles made of gold or silver are now virtually redundant since they require autoclaving and rapidly become blunt and painful to insert.

Other acupuncture microsystems

Apart from auricular acupuncture, several other systems that have been promoted use the concept of somatotopic representation, i.e. the body represented somewhere in miniature form, the homunculus. Inserting needles into the appropriate site is supposed to have an effect on the remote part, and in some cases the system is also used for diagnosis. The basis of these microsystems is actually a distortion of Sherington's original concept of the homunculus in the brain: he demonstrated that the body is represented on part of the cerebral cortex through somatotopically distributed neural connections.

New scalp acupuncture of Yamamoto

In Japan, Yamamoto developed a homunculus situated over the temple. This was a serendipitous finding: he was using acupuncture for treating various deficits in post-stroke patients, found he was wasting time waiting for patients to undress for body acupuncture, and hit on the idea of asking them just to remove their hats. In a busy clinic, this simple manoeuvre saves a good deal of time. Scalp acupuncture was already used for patients with stroke in some parts of China, usually involving threading a long needle subcutaneously over the affected area. Yamomoto evolved the idea that different points on the scalp represent different organs, reminiscent of Nogier's auricular charts. He extended the application of NSAY (new scalp acupuncture of Yamamoto) to other medical conditions, yet the therapy remains largely unevaluated.

Korean hand acupuncture

Korean hand acupuncture developed in 1971, and uses a slightly different idea: in this case, every meridian is supposed to be represented on the hands, including the conventionally named points. Treatment of the hands alone is supposed to be sufficient.

Interpretation

In summary, it seems possible that microsystems could be interpreted simply as an expression of the fact that needle treatment (almost) anywhere can produce valuable central effects, some specific and some non-specific. These effects rely on stimulating nerve endings, and the ear and hand are richly innervated. We have reservations about the microsystem concepts described here, and do not believe that the claims of somatotopic representation (i.e. body represented on one limited area) have been subjected to sufficient scrutiny in controlled trials.

Electrodiagnostic techniques

These techniques are quite distinct from EA treatment as described previously, which does not make any claims to diagnose patients.

Electroacupuncture after Voll

Voll was an electrical engineer who later studied biology and came across the concept of acupuncture points. While investigating their electrical properties, he developed an apparatus that could detect changes in skin resistance with pressure from a probe. The apparatus essentially consists of a Wheatstone bridge, but extra functions and sensitivities are claimed for it. In apparatus purchased on the open market, the circuitry is sealed with rubber to prevent examination. The EAV apparatus has stimulated many copies and 'developments', which add extra features and make additional claims. The makers of the apparatus claim it can measure the electrical performance of acupuncture points, which can be used to detect the underlying condition of individual organs of the body. A far as we are aware, the only rigorous investigation of this apparatus that has been carried out (testing how reliably it could detect allergies) was clearly negative (Lewith et al 2001).

Ryodoraku

In Japan in about 1950, Yosio Nakatani claimed to find a line of increased electroconductivity in the skin in meridians that related to diseased organs. Measurement of all the points, generally the terminal points on fingers and toes, is said to provide a diagnosis of the autonomic disturbance underlying the condition. Electrical stimulation at those points is given with the aim of correcting the disturbance.

Summary

It is wise to adopt a cautious approach toward novel treatments until they have been properly evaluated.

Continuous stimulation with indwelling needles may enhance the effectiveness of acupuncture in chronic pain, and indwelling studs can be used. The Japanese *umebari* technique involved inserting needles permanently, but has now been abandoned because of the trauma caused. Indwelling needles should be used with caution as they carry significant risks of infection, including local sepsis, bacteraemia and blood-borne spread of infection to another person if they fall out.

Auricular acupuncture developed in France, and the original principle was that the body is represented (upside down) on the auricle. There is no known mechanism for this idea; however, the auricle is well innervated and likely to be a good site for stimulating the central nervous system. The NADA technique is widely used for treatment of drug dependence. Continuous stimulation with studs has been used for smoking cessation, but because of the risks of indwelling needles in the ear, acupressure devices are now recommended.

Other stimulation techniques allied to acupuncture include acupressure, for example wristbands for treating nausea; moxibustion, which has limited use in a modern clinic; laser 'acupuncture' and transcutaneous electrical nerve stimulation (TENS). As these therapies do not involve needling, they have only a peripheral connection to acupuncture.

Other microsystems include new scalp acupuncture of Yamamoto (NSAY) and Korean hand acupuncture. Two electrodiagnostic techniques that involve some form of electrical measurement of acupuncture points are electroacupuncture after Voll (EAV), and Ryodoraku; these should be regarded as techniques that are completely distinct from electroacupuncture (EA).

SECTION 4 TREATMENT MANUAL

CHAPTER

15

Treatment guidelines

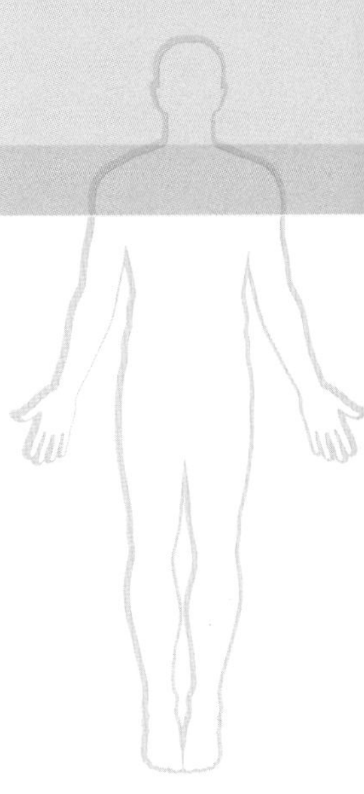

Contents

Introduction

This chapter should not be applied on its own, it is intended to be used only in the context of the particular approach to acupuncture that has been described in this book. Do not look here for formulae for treatment: there is no such thing as 'standardized' treatment, formula or prescription in acupuncture, any more than there is a standardized way to treat a respiratory infection – it all depends on the particular patient and their particular condition. You have discovered the principles of acupuncture in the previous chapters; here you will find some guidelines to point you in the right direction; the following chapter provides reference material to put these guidelines into practice. But it is still up to the acupuncturist to consider the actual patient and their individual case, and then to apply common sense and clinical judgement, in order to plan the best possible treatment. That is the art of medicine and also of acupuncture.

This chapter gives some guidelines on how to apply the principles to some common conditions. It is based, as always, on choosing the appropriate mechanism for the case. However, sometimes the cause of the clinical problem may not be clear-cut, and you may deliberately plan to combine several mechanisms. For example, you might choose a point because it has a local effect on the tissues as well as a segmental analgesic effect; or you might use a major point somewhere both for extrasegmental analgesia and for central regulatory effects.

Our guidelines are mostly about pain, and particularly musculoskeletal pain: this is both because pain is the condition that acupuncture is most commonly used for, and because in our experience it has the most predictable response, and the best understood mechanisms.

Although our approach to acupuncture is based on the current understanding of its mechanisms, there is still room for intuition. For example, you may decide to place a needle in a muscle tissue that is found to be tender, even though it might not be easy to link the location directly with the clinical picture. A therapeutic trial is justified as long as the patient is closely observed and the trial abandoned if there is no response within a reasonable time. This is not an excuse to think that acupuncture is just some kind of art form that relies entirely on intuition – the fundamental approach to the patient should always be based on a reasoned argument.

Finally, if you make a clinical observation that is novel or does not seem to fit into the current understanding, you are strongly encouraged to report it in the acupuncture literature as a case history. The rich tapestry of individual histories is fertile and challenging ground for helping to develop and extend our understanding of this ancient therapy.

Summary of general treatment principles

Selecting the point

By the time you have conducted the history and examination you will probably have formed a conclusion about the cause of the problem, and which of the five approaches the patient needs. Table 15.1 gives examples of the types

TABLE 15.1

Examples of conditions and point locations for different treatment approaches

Approach	Example of condition	Point location
Local	Local skin, or other soft tissue condition	Within about 25 mm of the problem, and about 20–50 mm apart
Segmental	Joint pain, other nociceptive pain; visceral conditions	In same segment, or adjacent segments; abdominal points for abdominal visceral conditions, paravertebral points for spinal conditions
Extrasegmental	Pain in several sites	Major points, bilaterally
Central regulatory	Pain with large affective component; conditions without pain	Major points, bilaterally
Myofascial trigger point (MTrP)	MTrP pain	Precisely on MTrP

of condition where the different mechanisms apply, and the sort of location where you may think about choosing points to needle.

Classical points can be chosen for needling because they are:

- myofascial trigger points
- tender points
- traditional acupuncture points.

Choose points that fit into more than one category if possible and, of course, you are not restricted to needling only classical points. However, only choose points that are in healthy tissue and have an intact nerve supply.

Stimulating the point

Stimulation is applied according to the type of mechanism that is to be activated, the nature of the patient and the patient's response. They are briefly summarized in Table 15.2.

Increasing the dose of treatment

Start with slight under-dosing, if anything, then increase the dose by:

- adding more points
- manipulating the needles for longer, and more than once
- possibly retaining the needles for longer (though from clinical observation the duration seems to make little difference)
- adding electroacupuncture (EA)
- adding another treatment approach, such as periosteal pecking or auricular acupuncture.

TABLE 15.2

Summary of methods of stimulation used in different treatment approaches

Approach	Stimulation
Local	Needle subcutaneously, and stimulate lightly
Segmental	Stimulate manually to elicit *de qi*, and maybe repeat stimulation at about 5- minute intervals; or use electroacupuncture; for 10–20 minutes; or periosteal pecking
Extrasegmental	Stimulate manually to elicit *de qi*, and preferably repeat at about 5- minute intervals; commonly use electroacupuncture for 10–30 minutes
Central regulatory	Gentle manual stimulation to elicit *de qi*, or sometimes electroacupuncture; 20–40 minutes leaving the patient to relax
Myofascial trigger point	Needle accurately to obtain local twitch responses; repeat if necessary, fanning out needle direction; or needle superficially; electroacupuncture may be useful for chronic MTrPs

Guidelines: musculoskeletal conditions

All guidelines are given with the usual caveat throughout this book. A standard medical diagnosis should be made in all patients before choosing acupuncture; acupuncture may relieve the symptoms of serious underlying disease temporarily and, thus, lead to delay in patients having the definitive treatment they need.

Myofascial trigger point pain

When the history suggests myofascial trigger point (MTrP) pain – unilateral pain that fluctuates, often for no obvious reason – identify the area of pain and compare it with the charts in the next chapter. Search across muscle fibres with your finger to find the MTrP, as described in detail in Chapter 7, and needle as is described in Chapter 12. Also, try to identify which activities provoke the pain and advise the patient to modify the way those exercises are performed or, if necessary, avoid them completely.

Osteoarthritis (OA)

- Start with a segmental approach using two to four local points including at least one traditional point and perhaps a tender point near the joint line
- Increase the dose by using more local segmental points and extrasegmental points – ideally, choose traditional points that are tender and are situated in the area of referred pain
- If you find active MTrPs in the muscles that act on the joint, treat them
- Periosteal pecking can be used in patients who appear less sensitive to needling or do not easily feel *de qi*, for example, on the greater trochanter for OA hip
- Do not insert needles into the joint space
- Do not expect complete relief in patients with serious joint destruction: there are finite limits to the potential of acupuncture, and it is no substitute for joint replacement surgery in advanced cases.

There follow some suggestions of traditional points that can be used to treat individual joints (see Chapter 16 for point locations):

- *Wrist* LU7
- *Base of thumb* LI4, TE5
- *Shoulder* LI15, SI11
- *Hip* GB30, GB29; distant segmental GB34
- *Knee* four local points including ST36, SP10, SP9; distant extrasegmental LR3
- *Ankle* BL60, KI3, LR3.

Spinal or paraspinal pain (neck, thorax, low back)

Try to localize the main level of origin of the pain by history and palpation, and to identify whether it is in the region of the spine or in the paravertebral tissues.

Examine for MTrPs that refer pain to the area, particularly in unilateral pain: they will most commonly be in trapezius for neck pain; rhomboids for thoracic pain; and erector spinae, quadratus lumborum or gluteus medius for pain in the lumbar region.

For spinal pain that is not due to MTrPs, use segmental points around the area of pain; mainly GV, *Huatuojiaji* and BL points, together with GB points in the neck and shoulders.

Reinforce or increase the effect by adding distant segmental or extrasegmental points, for example BL60.

Muscle spasm in patients with back pain can often be relieved swiftly by needling directly over or into the muscles involved, but this is likely to give only temporary relief if there is an underlying condition such as a prolapsed disc.

Soft-tissue conditions

Lateral epicondylitis

Consider this first as a symptom of MTrPs in the extensor muscles, and possibly supinator, and treat these in the usual way. If no MTrP can be found, or to increase the dose of treatment, use LI11, and add LI4 or periosteal pecking.

Medial epicondylitis

Similarly, search for MTrPs, but this time near the origin of the flexor group of muscles and pronator teres.

Shoulder pain

If pain is due to MTrPs arising from some episode when the muscles were overloaded, then acupuncture has a good chance of treating the pain successfully. However, classical 'frozen shoulder' is difficult to treat: the painful phase may be reduced in length, but it is not clear whether or not the time course of the restriction to the range of movement is reduced as well. EA is commonly used for chronic shoulder pain, and typical pairs of points would be LI15-LI16 and TE14-SI11.

Tenosynovitis, e.g. de Quervain's

Treat local tender points and acupuncture points, but do not needle the ligament sheath – avoid direct needling of any acutely inflamed tissue.

Plantar fasciitis

This condition can be difficult to treat with acupuncture, but occasionally the pain in the foot is due to an MTrP in the medial head of gastrocnemius: if so, you should be able to reproduce the patient's pain complaint by pressing over the TrP. For true plantar fasciitis, try local classical points; the plantar fascia itself is painful to needle, and the skin of the heel pad is thick and tough. However, it may be possible to needle directly into the tender point using a medial approach.

Ligaments and tendons

Soft-tissue injuries that are slow to recover can be encouraged to heal by brief needling, often at the most tender point. Acupuncture is likely to produce analgesia lasting some hours, so the patient should be warned not to overstretch the tissue (e.g. by playing sports) and thereby risk further injury.

Non-cardiac chest pain

If non-cardiac chest pain is not due to gastrointestinal disease, fibromyalgia or local conditions of the ribs, it is quite likely to be caused by MTrPs. Search for these in the pectoral muscles, mainly the pectoralis major, anywhere from the muscle attachment to the rib to the musculotendinous junction in the anterior axillary wall. Always beware of underlying lung – do not needle too deeply.

Guidelines: other painful conditions

Tension type headache

Examine the neck and shoulders for relevant MTrPs. These are likely to be found in the trapezii: these, and the posterior neck muscles and the suboccipital muscles should be examined systematically. In addition, the sternomastoids refer pain to the temporal and ear regions. Sometimes the history of the localization of the pain will enable you to diagnose which particular muscle harbours the MTrP, from the diagrams in the next chapter. Examine the neck in the sitting position, but treat the patient lying down: note that the MTrPs in postural muscles may not be so easy to find when lying down.

Commonly used traditional points for tension type headache are GB20 and GB21.

LI4 and LR3 are useful extrasegmental points for tension type headache, and may have central regulatory effects that could be beneficial if anxiety is prominent.

Migraine

The treatment of migraine involves finding and treating any relevant MTrPs in the neck and shoulders, and GB20, GB21, as for tension type headache, together with more emphasis on some major points for their central regulatory effect. Commonly used classical points are LR3 in particular and LI4.

Atypical facial pain

This may be due to undiagnosed MTrPs, so examine the masticatory muscles and the muscles of facial expression carefully; also consider primary MTrPs in upper trapezius. You may need to consult other texts for more detail on the pain referral patterns of individual muscles.

If no MTrPs can be found, then treatment should be directed to classical acupuncture points in the face together with GB20.

Fibromyalgia

Some patients clearly respond to acupuncture treatment so it is worth a trial. Temporary aggravations by acupuncture seem to be more common among patients with fibromyalgia than with other conditions, particularly from needling tender points in muscle – this is one condition where practitioners should be cautious of treating tender points (another is complex regional pain syndrome).

The wisest approach is to use gentle treatment initially on some major points in hands and feet, and, if possible, some points near the symptoms, but only if they are not too tender. Some authorities recommend only 30 seconds treatment with each needle. If this is enough to start a response, then this can be reinforced by gradually leaving the needles in place for longer. However, if there is no strong reaction to the first treatment, it is probably best to use EA – the present evidence suggests that this will be most beneficial.

Patients with fibromyalgia often have one or two distinct areas of myofascial pain as well as the generalized soft-tissue pain. It is thought that targeting this myofascial pain may not only improve the localized pain, but may result in some general improvement in the condition. Treatment should be cautious initially since compliance will be reduced if post-needling soreness is excessive.

Intermittent claudication

Use the traditional points BL57 and major points on the feet, as well as any TrPs in the gastrocnemius and soleus muscles, and segmental points at L2 level. Any improvement in the condition is likely to be through reducing secondary myofascial pain rather than improved circulation.

Be aware that this condition tends to improve spontaneously somewhat in the period after first diagnosis, so do not be overeager in claiming to have cured the patient!

Phantom limb pain

Check for trigger points on the stump, and treat them cautiously because of the risk of painful reaction. You can also use classical points in the residual limb or limb girdle, and paravertebral points on the same side.

Treat mirror points on the other limb – mirror images of the points in the area of pain – and consider auricular acupuncture.

Trigeminal or post-herpetic neuralgia

Treat the segment above (or below) the affected segment, or the segment on the opposite side (mirror points), for fear of a painful reaction to needling the affected segment. You may need to add EA.

If there is no response, then treat within the segment, but only gently at first.

Complex regional pain syndrome and Raynaud's syndrome

Though the pathology of these two conditions is clearly different, they can be approached in a similar way, and a few patients with each condition will respond.

Choose local major points in the affected limb and limb girdle, but do not give strong treatment to sensitive sites, for fear of aggravating the symptoms.

Add paraspinal segmental needling to the relevant segments (see Fig. 16.14) to influence the sympathetic outflow.

Guidelines: abdominal symptoms

Gastrointestinal symptoms

Acupuncture will mainly be symptomatic, directed to the relief of pain and dysfunction in conditions such as irritable bowel syndrome. The simplest and most effective approach is to needle tender points in the abdominal wall muscles (segmental approach) or strong abdominal points, such as CV12 and ST25. Major points in the lower limb, such as ST36, LR3, will have extrasegmental and central regulatory effects.

Bladder symptoms

As above, needle the tender points over the lower abdominal wall for any bladder symptoms, such as irritative bladder. Add points over the sacrum (BL points) and several lumbar paravertebral points for the autonomic outflow, and pick up the sacral segments in the lower limb, e.g. SP6, ST36, LR3. See also Tables 16.1 and 16.2.

Guidelines: conditions without pain

Nausea

Nausea due to pregnancy, surgery or chemotherapy can often be diminished by treatment with acupuncture, typically PC6 and possibly ST36, although needle location may not be critical. Ideally, start the treatment before the onset of nausea. Unlike when treating pain, the relief of nausea does not seem to last more than a day or so; patients should either be treated quite frequently, say three times a week, or shown how to use acupressure bands, which they should massage 2 hourly.

Hayfever, allergic rhinitis

Typical points used are LI20, *Yintang*, *Taiyang* together with LI11 and ST36. Add LI4 and LR3 if needed to increase the dose.

Acupuncture may give instant relief for hayfever, presumably due to a sympathetic response; and if repeated weekly about three times before the season it may prevent attacks altogether.

Menopausal hot flushes

Any general stimulation is likely to produce a response, typically LI4, SP6 and LR3. EA may have some benefit over manual needling.

Tinnitus

Tinnitus may occasionally be a symptom of an MTrP deep in the masseter muscle – a likely clue is that the symptoms will fluctuate, and are likely to be unilateral and not associated with hearing loss. Persistent, continuous tinnitus has occasionally appeared to respond to local needling at SI19, GB20, etc., but RCTs have not shown specific effects.

Itch

Sometimes pruritus responds to acupuncture – local needles surrounding any particular lesion and the usual major points for an overall effect.

Safety first

We shall not repeat the advice on safe practice in other chapters of this book, but simply remind readers that they must constantly think of the patient's safety as well as the effectiveness of the acupuncture treatment.

Recording treatment

Records of treatment need to be as precise as possible, within the limits of the space available in clinical notes, indicating the points used, the amount of stimulation and the duration of needle retention. It is important to know what you have done at one treatment, so you can adjust it next time according to the response – which should also be diligently recorded especially after the initial treatment.

Some standard symbols can be used as a kind of shorthand, as shown in Table 15.3. The points used can be written (or a small diagram if not a known

TABLE 15.3

Examples of records of acupuncture treatment

Treatment details	Shorthand record in notes
One needle inserted superficially at LI11 without stimulation, retained for 5 minutes	LI11 S1 x0–5′
Treatment of these four major points with deep needles given one stimulation and retained for 20 minutes	LI4, LR3 D4 x1–20′
Moderately strong manual needling at three points, retained for 20 minutes	ST36, SP9, SP10 D3 x2–20′
Strong periosteal needling to one point for 10 seconds (describe the point, e.g. tip of acromion, or draw small diagram)	P1 x3 –10″
Electroacupuncture given at stated frequencies, for 30 minutes (drawing indicates location)	EA 4/80Hz–30′

point) with two circles above for bilateral treatment, and the letter R or L for unilateral treatment; some kind of scale such as x0 to x3 to indicate the amount of manual stimulation, using P for periosteal needling, EA for electroacupuncture; and the duration of needle retention, in minutes.

CHAPTER

16

Reference charts: points and innervation

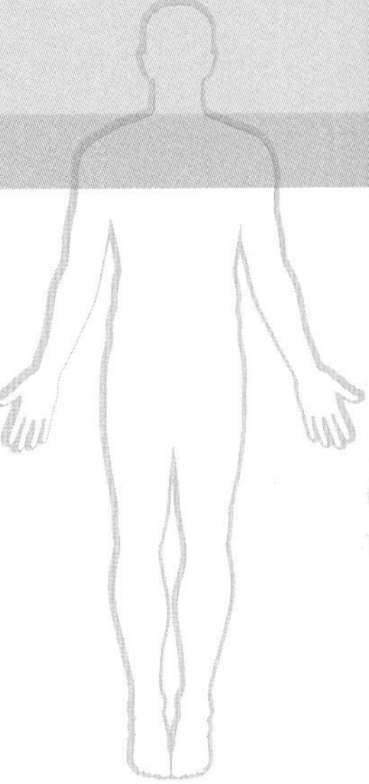

Contents

How to locate acupuncture points

Myofascial trigger point pain referral patterns

Ask the patient to delineate the area of their pain as precisely as possible, then look for the pattern on the appropriate chart. Myofascial trigger point (MTrP) diagrams include the site of the MTrP indicated with a cross-hatch symbol. The long strokes of the symbol indicate the muscle fibre orientation. The two-tone shaded areas are examples of possible pain referral patterns from the relevant TrPs. The darker areas indicate the more frequent sites of pain. Prepare your acupuncture needle so you can immediately treat any point(s) you find.

Feel the fibres under the fingertips, feeling for the taut band then for the most tender part of the taut band. Most muscles can be examined by flat palpation. Use pincer palpation for the anterior border of trapezius in the shoulder in slim individuals, the lateral fibres of the pectoralis major in the anterior axillary wall and the sternomastoid (gently).

Traditional acupuncture points

We have chosen a sample of points for this introductory book because they are either:

- major points for extrasegmental acupuncture or central regulatory effects: LI4, TE5, PC6, LI11, ST36, SP6, KI3, BL60, LR3, or
- useful in treating common conditions (round arthritic joints), or

- illustrative of principles of locating points elsewhere (alongside the spine), or
- at or close to common myofascial trigger points (e.g. GB21).

Readers who want to learn more traditional points (instead of using their fingers to find appropriate places to treat) can look in the texts listed at the end of this chapter.

Bony landmarks

Classical points tend to be either dips into which the finger sinks naturally (ST36), or at the summit of a prominence, for example a bulging muscle (LI4). They often are described in relation to a particular skin crease or to a bony landmark – the prominence of the spinous processes, a joint line, the highest point of the femoral tuberosity. For those unfamiliar with superficial anatomy, we add some aides memoire for identifying individual locations, where appropriate.

Find the actual point for inserting the needle by exploring with the finger for the most tender site. Myofascial trigger points need to be located by the special technique described in Chapter 7.

Body measurements

The Chinese system of proportional measurement is still useful for finding some of the points. The Chinese argued that patients do not come in fixed sizes, so they divided each part of the body into a constant number of units. They called the unit *cun* (pronounced tsun), which is sometimes referred to as the 'Chinese inch'. For example, the middle phalanx of the middle finger is one *cun*, and the elbow crease to the wrist crease is 12 *cun* (Fig. 16.1). Points are best found by subdividing up the whole distance, but an alternative is to count *cun* from one end.

Conveniently, the fingers can be used in various combinations to make measurements (Fig. 16.2). For example, one important point, PC6 is located 2 *cun* up from the wrist. Although obviously it should be the patient's own hand that is used, in practice it is the examiner's hand that is often used after a quick comparison with that of the patient – which is fine because points really do not have to be located all that precisely.

Most points are found by measuring from a bony landmark using the fingers; but the abdomen is usually measured, at least in the axial direction, by using the fixed divisions or *cun*.

Acupuncture points by region

In Figures 16.4–16.13, we present the points by region. Descriptions of the points are given, together with notes on locating them where relevant, and some conditions they are commonly used for. Also listed is the innervation of the dermatome (D), myotome (M) and sclerotome (S) where this information is relevant clinically. When the point's sclerotome is not applicable, e.g.

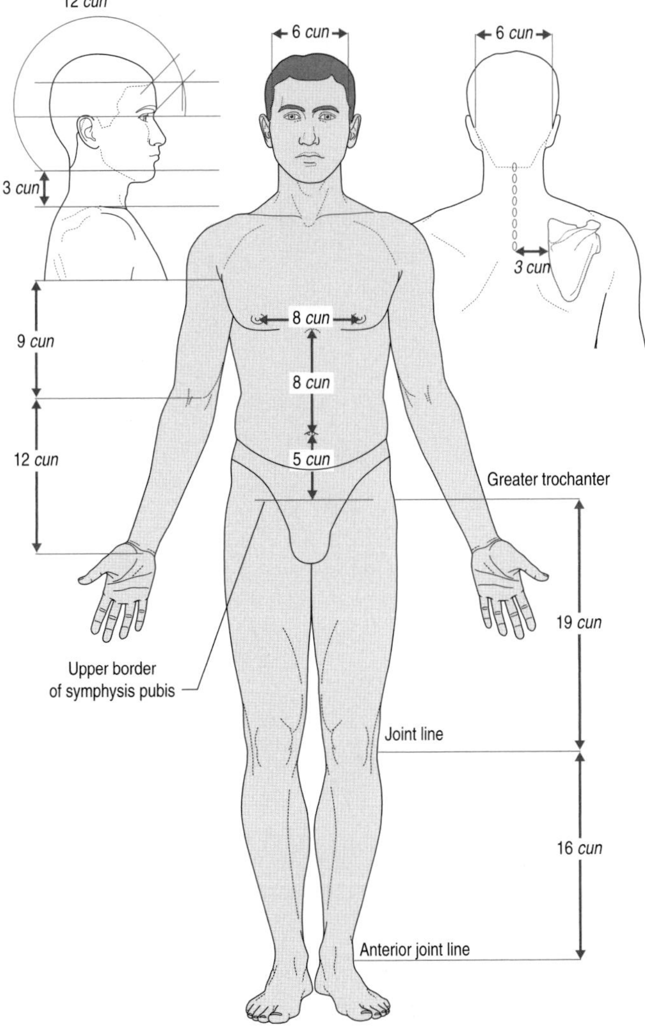

Figure 16.1 Proportional measurement of various parts of the body.

because the periosteum is not accessible, no level is given. Where a point clearly relates to a single MTrP, the relevant muscle is named.

Needling direction can be assumed to be perpendicular unless stated otherwise.

The site of the MTrP is indicated with a cross-hatch symbol (rather than the usual X in other texts) so that the long strokes of the symbol indicate the muscle fibre orientation (Fig. 16.3). The two-tone shaded areas are examples of possible pain referral patterns from each MTrP, the darker areas indicating more common sites of pain.

An exclamation mark (!) against a point or directions for use indicates a particular risk. No needle should be inserted without first considering whether the local anatomy presents risks to treatment.

Clinical conditions for which the point is commonly used are listed (Figs 16.4–16.13).

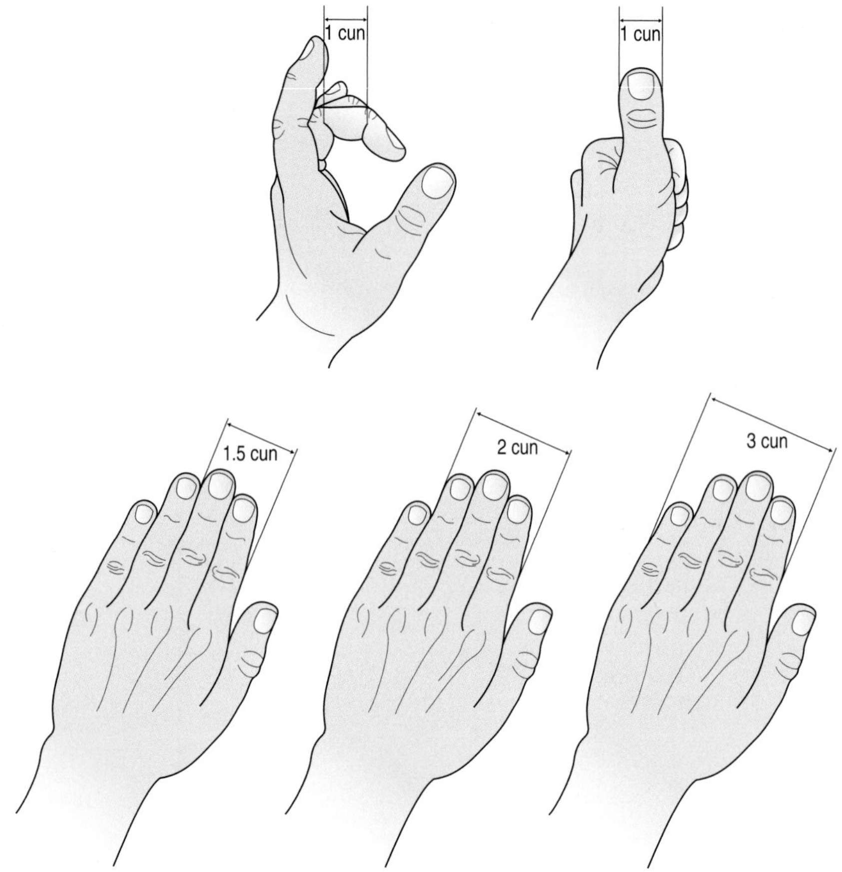

Figure 16.2 Use of the fingers and thumb to measure one, two and three cun.

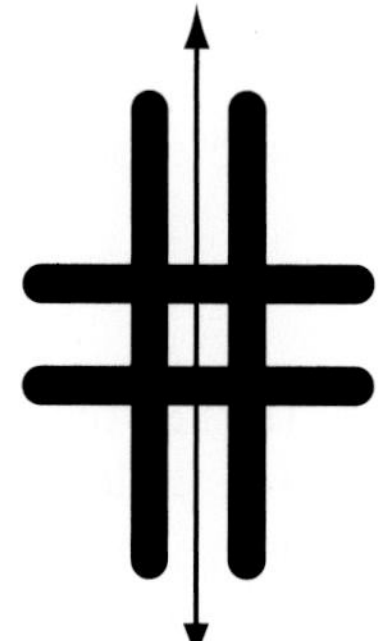

Figure 16.3 Cross-hatch symbol used to indicate the trigger point, the longitudinal strokes indicating the muscle fibre orientation.

Other reference tables

Table 16.2 shows segmental levels of the autonomic innervation of the body.

Table 16.3 shows spinal segmental levels and their relationship to acupuncture points.

Figure 16.14 shows the dermatomes of the back.

Table 16.4 shows some common sites for periosteal pecking that are accessible and generally safe.

Clinical observations suggest that the points shown in Table 16.5 are likely to be particularly useful for extrasegmental analgesic effects and central regulatory effects. They appear repeatedly in the formulae for treatment of a wide range of conditions, usually treated bilaterally.

Since there is no evidence that the meridians have any structure or function, there seems little point in learning their pathways in detail. They can be useful insofar as they act as *aides memoire* for the acupuncture points. Figures 16.15 and 16.16, and Tables 16.6 and 16.7 show what we think may be helpful or relevant to medical acupuncturists. Note that we present the meridians in the traditional order simply by convention.

Further reading

Baldry P E 2005 Acupuncture, trigger points and musculoskeletal pain. Elsevier Ltd, Edinburgh

The illustrations and figures in this book will be particularly useful to acupuncturists who want to develop their knowledge and skill in treating myofascial pain.

Campbell A 2001 Acupuncture in practice: beyond points and meridians. Butterworth-Heinemann, Oxford

Anthony Campbell describes a rational approach to treatment that he has developed from the traditional practice, using 'acupuncture treatment areas'. This book explains how to apply this approach throughout the body.

Hecker H-U, Steveling A, Peuker E et al 2001 Color atlas of acupuncture. Thieme, Stuttgart

This book is a model of clarity for anyone who wants exact descriptions of a selection of acupuncture points. However, it is full of traditional Chinese theory! It includes sections on body points, auricular points and myofascial trigger points.

Mann F 1992 Reinventing acupuncture. Butterworth-Heinemann, Oxford

Felix Mann describes his approach to treatment in detail, which is based on his observations and anatomical knowledge. He uses treatment areas rather than traditional points, and his approach is based on clinical experience not physiological mechanisms.

FIGURE 16.4

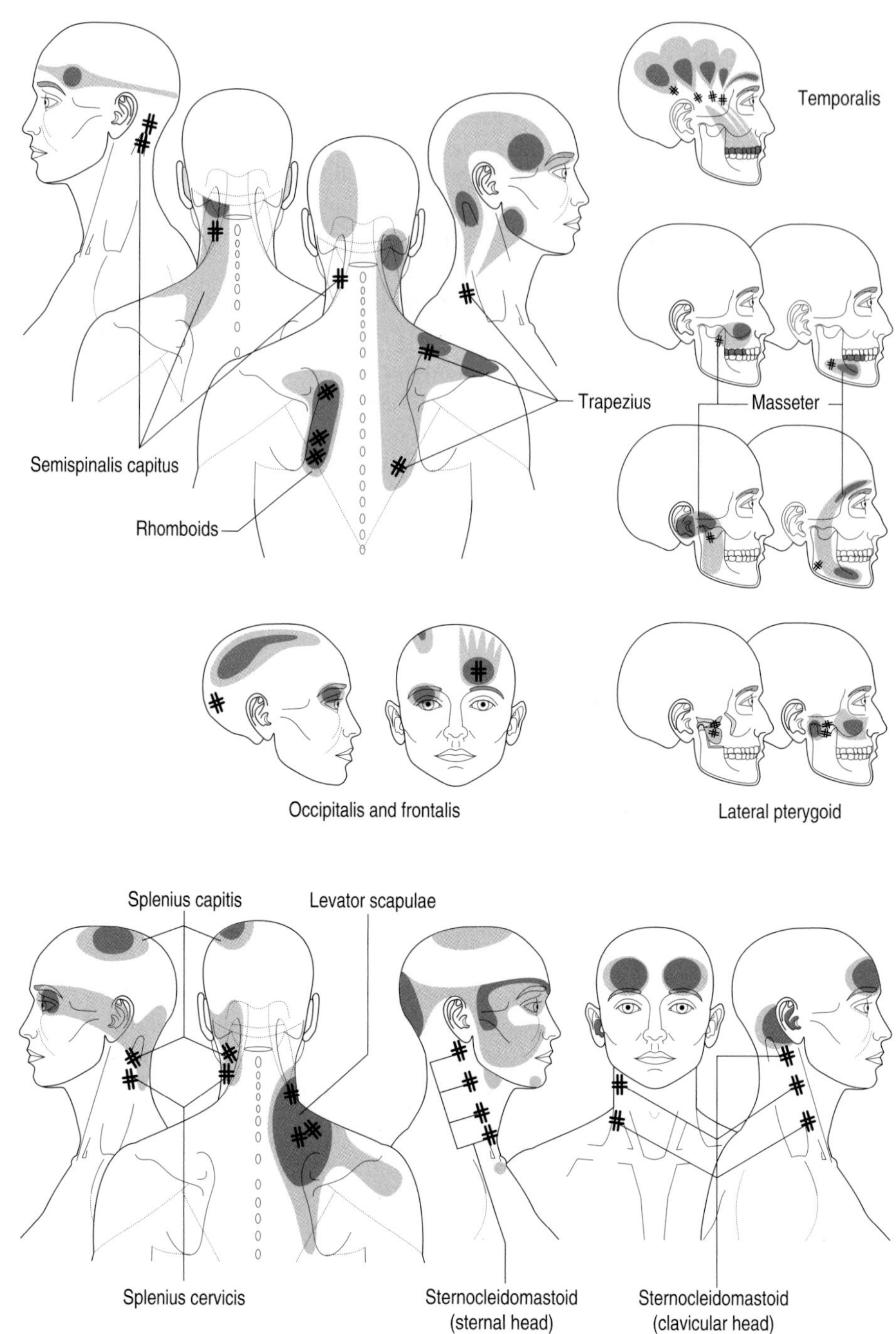

Figure 16.4 Head, face and neck: myofascial trigger points and pain reference zones.

FIGURE 16.5

Figure 16.5 Head, face and neck: classical acupuncture points and trigger points.

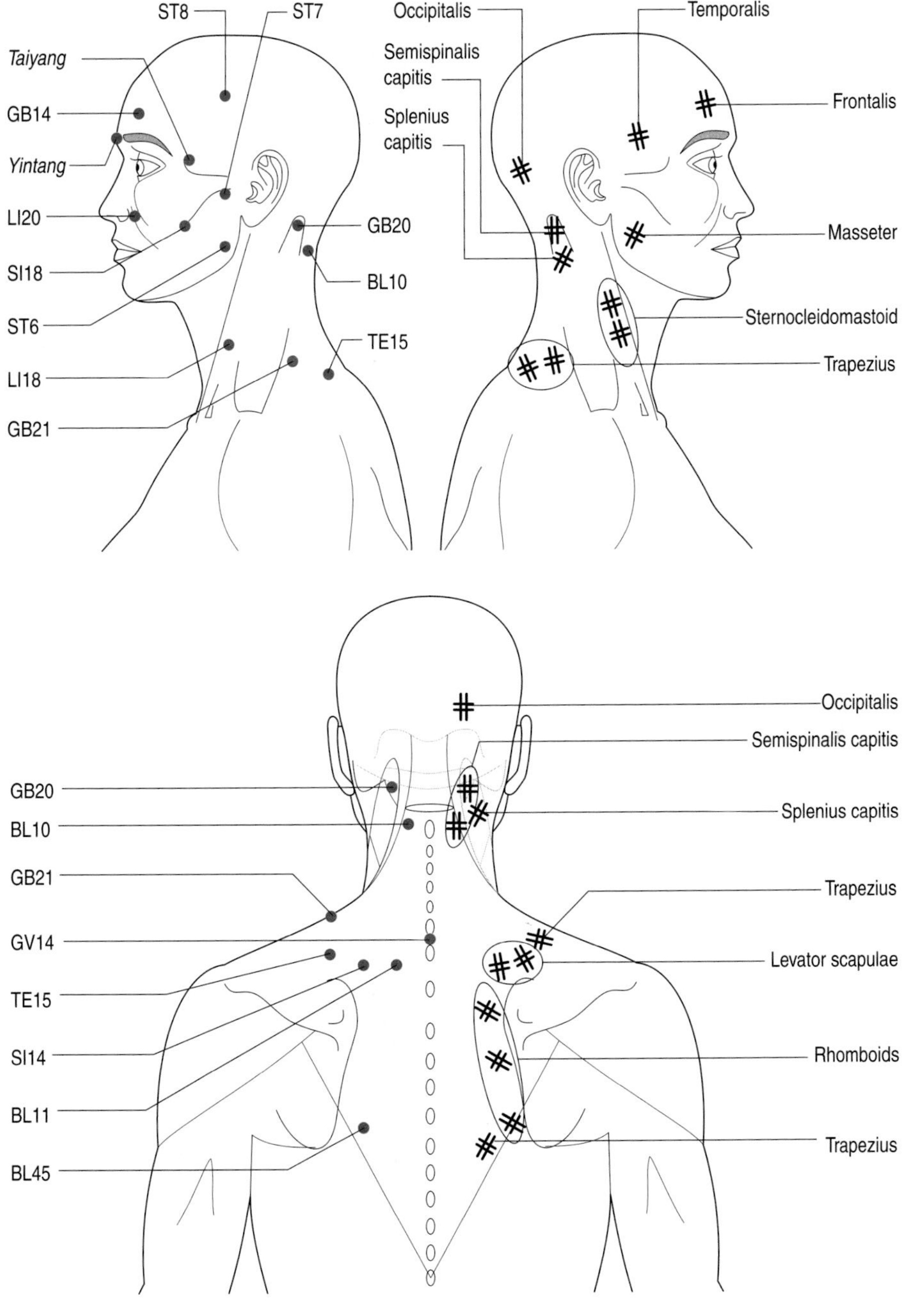

TABLE 16.1.1

Table 16.1.1 Head, face and neck

Face		
Yintang	Midpoint between the eyebrows **Angulation:** oblique inferior **Target:** procerus or periosteum *Headache, hayfever, relaxation*	D Vi M VII S Vi
Taiyang	1 *cun* posterior to the midpoint between the lateral end of the eyebrow and the lateral canthus of the eye **Angulation:** perpendicular **Target:** temporalis *Headache, eye symptoms*	D Vii M Viii S Vii
GB14	1 *cun* above the middle of the eyebrow, directly above the pupil when the eyes are looking straight ahead **Angulation:** oblique inferior **Target:** frontalis *Headache, eye symptoms*	D Vi M VII S Vi
LI20	In the nasolabial groove, level with the widest part of the ala nasi **Angulation:** superiorly along groove **Target:** facial muscles *Hayfever, nasal symptoms*	D Vii M VII S Vii
ST6	1 fingerbreadth anterior and superior to the angle of the jaw, on the prominence of masseter **Angulation:** perpendicular **Target:** masseter *Dental pain, facial pain*	D C2/C3 M Viii S Viii
ST7	In the depression anterior to the temporomandibular joint and below the zygomatic arch **Angulation:** perpendicular **Target:** lateral pterygoid *Dental pain, facial pain*	D Viii M Viii S Viii
ST8	0.5 *cun* superior to the upper line of origin of the temporalis muscle, directly above ST7 and ST6 on a vertical line 0.5 cun posterior to Taiyang **Angulation:** perpendicular **Target:** epicranial tissues *Headache*	D Vi/Vii M Viii/VII S Vi/Vii
SI18	Directly below the lateral canthus of the eye in the depression at the lower border of the zygomatic bone, just anterior to the attachment of masseter **Angulation:** slightly superior **Target:** connective tissue space *Facial pain, trigeminal neuralgia*	D Vii M Viii S Vii
LI18	Between the sternal and clavicular heads of sternocleidomastoid (SCM), level with the laryngeal prominence (the tip of the Adam's apple) **Angulation:** posterior **Target:** fascial plane in SCM *Pain from sternocleidomastoid – headache or facial pain* **CAUTION – note the proximity of the carotid artery**	D C2/C3 M XI/C2/C3 S n/a

D = dermatome, M = myotome, S = sclerotome, V = trigeminal nerve, i = ophthalmic, ii = maxillary, iii = mandibular divisions, VII = facial nerve, XI = accessory nerve, n/a = not applicable

Meridian abbreviations – see Tables 16.6 and 16.7, page 218.

Head and neck

Point	Location / angulation / target / indications	Innervation
GB20	Below the occipital bone, in the depression between trapezius and sternomastoid and above splenius capitis **Angulation:** towards opposite eyebrow **Target:** semispinalis capitis *Headache, neck pain and stiffness* **CAUTION – note the position of the vertebral artery**	D C2/C3 M C1/C2 S C1/C2
BL10	1.3 *cun* lateral to the spinous process of C2, between C1 and C2 **Angulation:** towards lamina of C2 **Target:** obliquus inferior *Neck pain and stiffness* **CAUTION – note the position and depth of the spinal cord and vertebral artery**	D C3 M C1 to C5 S C2/C3
GB21	Midway between GV14 and tip of the acromion at the highest point of trapezius **Angulation:** tangential to ribs, posteriorly **Target:** upper trapezius *Headache, neck pain and stiffness, anxiety* **CAUTION – note the proximity of the pleura between the 1st and 2nd ribs**	D C3 M C3/C4 S n/a
TE15	Midway between the points GB21 and SI13 at the superior angle of the Scapula (SI13 – tender depression superior to medial end of scapular spine) **Angulation:** perpendicular **Target:** trapezius *Shoulder pain, neck pain and stiffness* **CAUTION – note the proximity of the pleura in slim patients**	D C3 M C3/C4 S n/a
GV14	Between spinous processes C7 and T1 **Angulation:** transverse **Target:** interspinous ligament *Spinal neck pain, headache of cervical origin*	D C4/C5/T1 M C8 S C8
SI14	3 *cun* lateral to spinous process of T1 **Angulation:** tangential towards scapula **Target:** levator scapulae *Shoulder pain, neck pain and stiffness* **CAUTION – do not needle deeply unless confident of angulation relative to scapula**	D C3/C4 M C3/C4/C5 S C5
BL11	1.5 *cun* lateral to the lower border of the spinous process of T1 **Angulation:** oblique towards spine **Target:** rhomboid minor *Neck pain and stiffness, dyspnoea* **CAUTION – do not needle deeply unless confident of angulation relative to pleura**	D C4/T1 M C4/C5 S T1/T2
BL45	3 *cun* lateral to the lower border of the spinous process of T6 **Angulation:** oblique towards spine **Target:** iliocostalis thoracis *Dorsal back pain, dyspnoea* **CAUTION – do not needle deeply unless confident of angulation relative to pleura**	D T5/T6 M T6/T7 S T6/T7

FIGURE 16.6

Figure 16.6 Shoulder and arm: myofascial trigger points and pain reference zones.

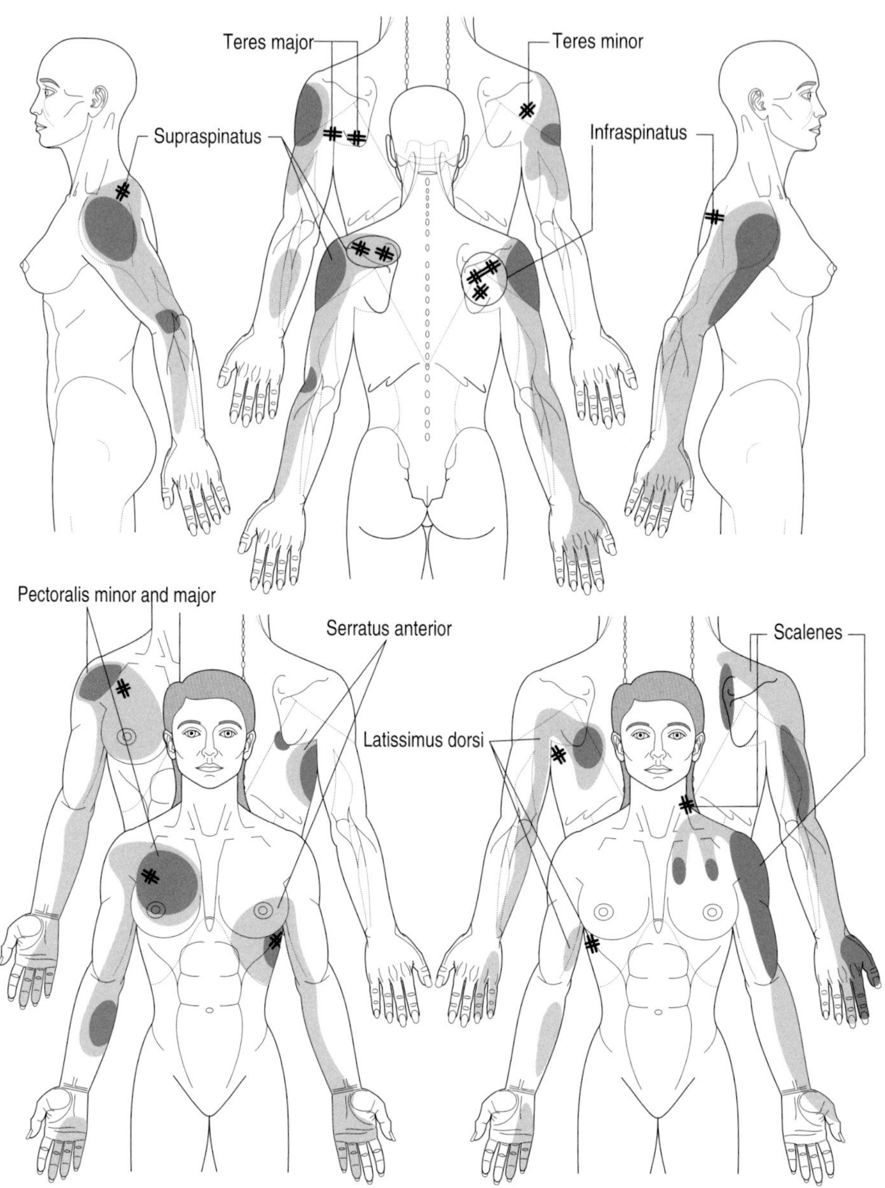

FIGURE 16.7

Figure 16.7 Shoulder and arm: classical acupuncture points and trigger points.

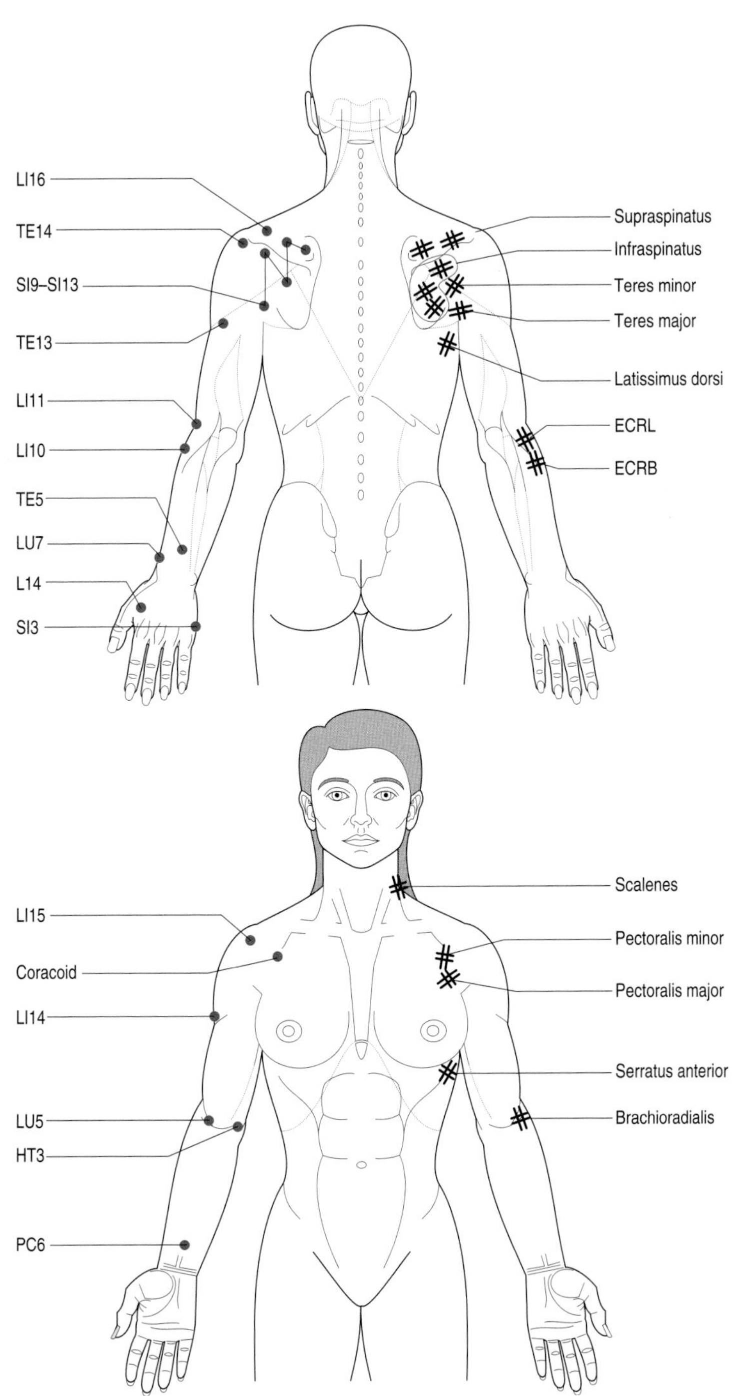

TABLE 16.1.2

Table 16.1.2 Shoulder and arm

Posterior aspect		
LI16	In the depression medial to the acromion and between the lateral extremities of the clavicle and scapular spine **Angulation:** perpendicular **Target:** supraspinatus *Shoulder and arm pain*	D C3 M C3 to C6 S C5/C6
TE14	Posterolateral and inferior to the posterior tip of the acromion, in the depression between the middle and posterior fibres of deltoid **Angulation:** perpendicular **Target:** infraspinatus insertion *Shoulder and arm pain*	D C3/C4 M C5/C6 S C6
SI9	1 *cun* superior to the posterior axillary crease when the arm hangs by the side of the body **Angulation:** perpendicular **Target:** teres major *Shoulder and arm pain*	D T3/T4 M C5/C6/C7 S C7
SI10	In the depression below the spine of the scapula, directly superior to the posterior axillary crease when the arm hangs by the side of the body **Angulation:** perpendicular **Target:** infraspinatus *Shoulder and arm pain*	D C3/C4 M C5/C6 S C6
SI11	1/3 down a line from the midpoint of the scapular spine to the inferior angle of the scapula **Angulation:** perpendicular **Target:** infraspinatus *Shoulder and arm pain*	D C4/T1/T2 M C5/C6 S C5/C6
SI12	Directly above SI11 in the middle of the suprascapular fossa, about 1 *cun* above the middle of the superior border of the scapular spine **Angulation:** towards suprascapular fossa **Target:** supraspinatus *Shoulder and arm pain* **CAUTION – do not needle deeply unless confident of position relative to scapula**	D C3/C4 M C3 to C6 S C5
SI13	In the tender depression superior to the medial end of the scapular spine **Angulation:** towards suprascapular fossa **Target:** supraspinatus *Shoulder and arm pain* **CAUTION – do not needle deeply unless confident of position relative to scapula**	D C4/T1 M C3 to C6 S C5
TE13	On the line connecting the olecranon and TE14, 3 *cun* distal to TE14 on the posterior border of deltoid, 2 *cun* lateral to the posterior axillary fold **Angulation:** perpendicular **Target:** lateral head of triceps *Shoulder and arm pain* **CAUTION – note the proximity of the radial nerve**	D C5 M C6/C7/C8 S C6/C7
LI11	At the radial end of the antecubital crease, halfway between the biceps tendon and the lateral epicondyle **Angulation:** perpendicular **Target:** extensor carpi radialis longus *Lateral epicondylalgia, forearm pain; immunomodulation*	D C5/C6 M C5/C6 S C6/C7
LI10	2 *cun* distal to LI11, on the line connecting LI11 with LI5 (the centre of the anatomical snuff box) **Angulation:** perpendicular **Target:** extensor carpi radialis longus or supinator *Lateral epicondylalgia, forearm pain*	D C5/C6 M C5/C6/C7 S C6/C7

D = dermatome, M = myotome, S = sclerotome, n/a = not applicable

Meridian abbreviations – see Tables 16.6 and 16.7, page 218.

Posterior aspect

TE5	On the dorsal surface of forearm, 2 *cun* proximal to wrist joint, between radius and ulna, and between extensor indicis and extensor pollicis longus **Angulation:** perpendicular **Target:** connective tissue plane *Local pain; wrist and forearm; major point for central effects*	D C6 to C8 M C7/C8 S C7/C8
LU7	On the radial aspect of the radial styloid, 1.5 *cun* from the wrist crease, between the tendons of abductor pollicis longus and brachioradialis **Angulation:** proximal oblique **Target:** connective tissue space *Wrist and forearm pain*	D C6 M C7/C8 S C6
LI4	On the dorsal aspect of the hand, in the middle of the 1st web space, halfway along the second metacarpal bone **Angulation:** perpendicular **Target:** 1st dorsal interosseous *General point for pain; major point for central effects* **CAUTION – the radial artery is at the apex of the 1st web space**	D C6/C7 M T1 S n/a
SI3	On the palmar aspect of the neck of the 5th metacarpal, in the tissue plane between the metacarpal neck and the hypothenar muscles **Angulation:** perpendicular **Target:** connective tissue plane *Hand pain; also used for pain elsewhere especially spinal pain*	D C8 M T1 S C8

Anterior aspect

LI15	Anterolateral and inferior to the anterior tip of the acromion, in the groove between the anterior and middle fibres of deltoid **Angulation:** perpendicular **Target:** supraspinatus insertion *Shoulder and arm pain*	D C4 M C5 S C5
Coracoid	Anterior to the glenohumeral joint, between the fibres of deltoid and pectoralis major **Angulation:** perpendicular **Target:** coracoid *Shoulder and arm pain*	D C4 M C5/C6 S C5
LI14	Between the distal attachment of deltoid and the long head of biceps, in a tender depression, 3/5 of the distance on a line from LI11 to LI15 **Angulation:** perpendicular **Target:** connective tissue plane *Shoulder and arm pain*	D C5/C6 M C5/C6 S C5/C6
LU5	On the cubital crease of the elbow, in the depression on the radial side of the biceps tendon **Angulation:** perpendicular **Target:** brachioradialis *Elbow or forearm pain*	D C5/C6 M C5/C6 S C5/C6
HT3	At the medial end of the antecubital crease when the elbow is fully flexed **Angulation:** perpendicular **Target:** pronator teres *Medial epicondylalgia, forearm pain* **CAUTION – note the proximity of the brachial artery**	D T1 M C5 to T1 S C7
PC6	2 *cun* proximal to the distal wrist crease, between the tendons of flexor carpi radialis and palmaris longus **Angulation:** oblique proximal **Target:** flexor digitorum superficialis *Nausea and vomiting, carpal tunnel syndrome* **CAUTION – note the position of the median nerve directly below**	D C6/C8/T1 M C7/C8 S n/a

FIGURE 16.8

Figure 16.8 Thorax and abdomen: myofascial trigger points and pain reference zones.

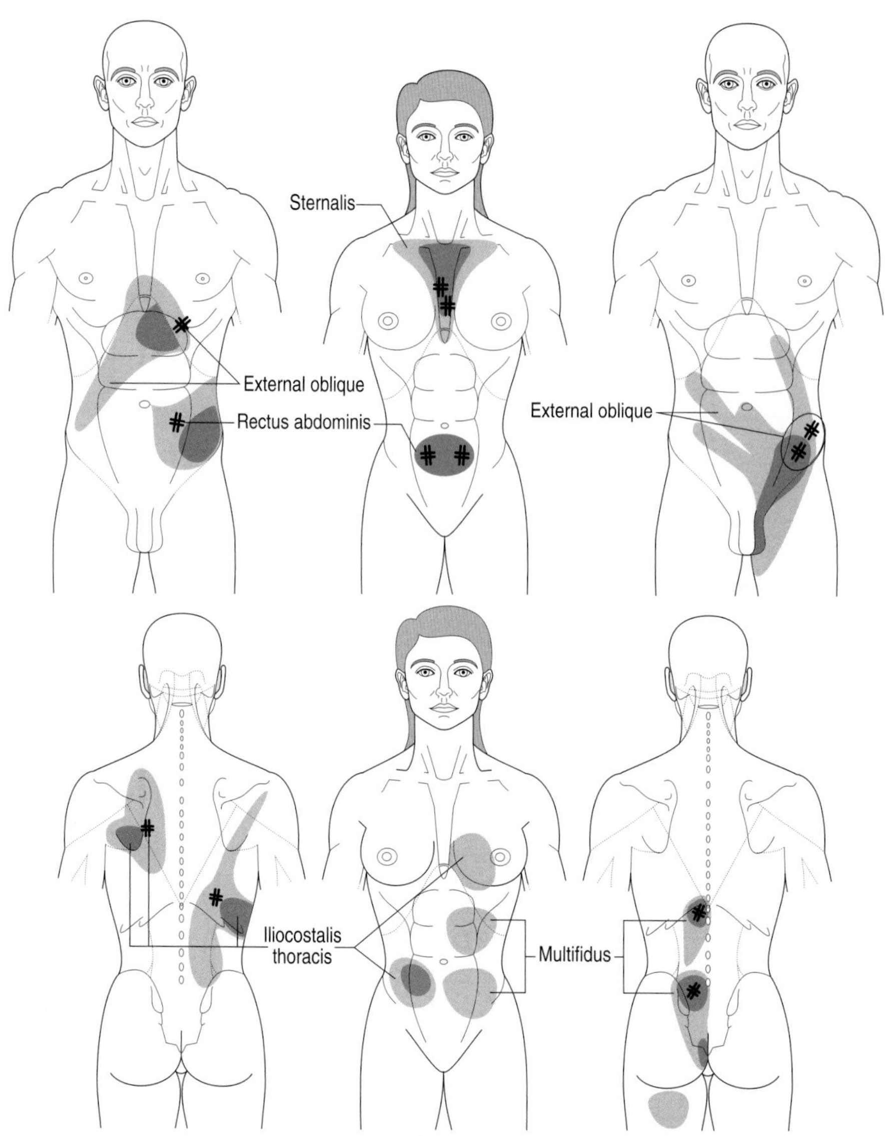

FIGURE 16.9

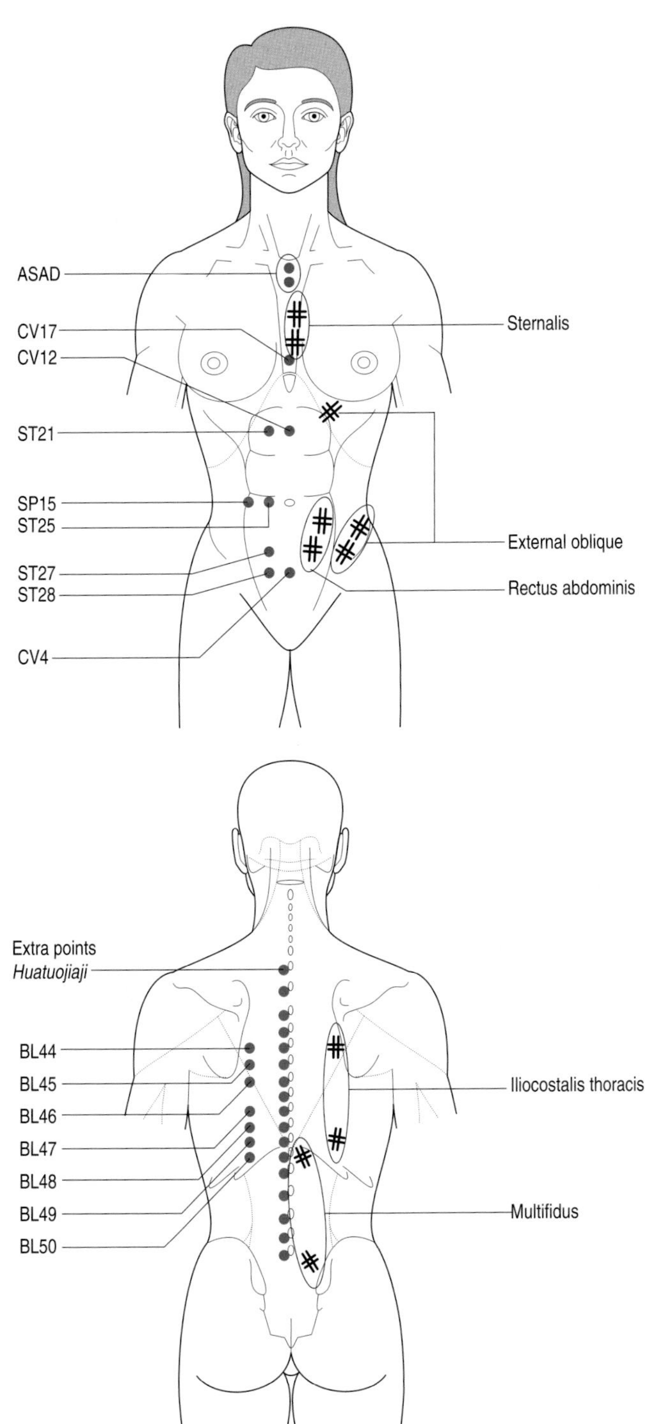

Figure 16.9 Thorax, abdomen and spine: classical acupuncture points and trigger points.

TABLE 16.1.3

Table 16.1.3 Thorax and abdomen

Anterior aspect		
ASAD	Two points in the midline just below the sternal notch over the manubrium **Angulation:** perpendicular **Target:** periosteum of manubrium *Anxiety, sickness and dyspnoea*	D C4/T2 M C5/C6 S T1
CV17	In the center of the sternum at the 4th intercostal space (level with nipples in a man) **Angulation:** cranial oblique at 30 degrees to the sternum **Target:** periosteum of the sternum or sternalis *Chest pain; respiratory conditions* **CAUTION – a sternal foramen occurs at this point in 10% of men and 4% of women; never needle perpendicularly**	D T5 M C8, T1 S T1
CV12	On the midline of the upper abdomen, midway between the umbilicus and the lower border of the body of the sternum **Angulation:** perpendicular **Target:** linea alba *Upper gastrointestinal disorders, including nausea and vomiting* **CAUTION – avoid needling through the abdominal wall**	D T8 M T8 S n/a
CV4	On the midline of the lower abdomen, 3 *cun* inferior to the umbilicus, and 2 *cun* superior to the pubic symphysis **Angulation:** perpendicular **Target:** linea alba *Lower gastrointestinal, urological and gynaecological symptoms* **CAUTION – avoid needling through the abdominal wall**	D T11/T12 M T11/T12 S n/a
SP15	At the lateral border of rectus abdominis level with the umbilicus **Angulation:** perpendicular **Target:** linea semilunaris *Abdominal pain* **CAUTION – avoid needling through the abdominal wall**	D T10/T11 M T10/T11 S n/a
Kidney and Stomach meridians run parallel with CV with points over the abdomen at most segments – any tender point can be treated		
ST21	2 *cun* lateral to CV12 **Angulation:** medial oblique [non-classical] **Target:** rectus abdominis *Upper abdominal pain; gastroenterological symptoms* **CAUTION – avoid needling through the abdominal wall**	D T7/T8 M T7/T8 S n/a
ST25	2 *cun* lateral to the umbilicus, halfway between the umbilicus and the linea semilunaris (SP15) **Angulation:** perpendicular **Target:** rectus abdominis *Abdominal pain; gastroenterological symptoms* **CAUTION – avoid needling through the abdominal wall**	D T10 M T10 S n/a
ST27	2 *cun* lateral to the midline and 2 *cun* inferior to the umbilicus **Angulation:** medial oblique [non-classical] **Target:** rectus abdominis *Abdominal pain; lower gastrointestinal, urological and gynaecological symptoms* **CAUTION – avoid needling through the abdominal wall**	D T11/T12 M T11/T12 S n/a
ST28	2 *cun* lateral to the midline and 3 *cun* inferior to the umbilicus **Angulation:** medial oblique [non-classical] **Target:** rectus abdominis *Abdominal pain; lower gastrointestinal, urological*	D T12/L1 M T12/L1 S n/a

D = dermatome, M = myotome, S = sclerotome, n/a = not applicable

Meridian abbreviations – see Tables 16.6 and 16.7, page 218.

Posterior aspect

Huatuojiaji	A series of 17 extra points, 0.5 *cun* lateral to the lower border of the spinous processes of T1 to L5 **Angulation:** oblique towards spine **Target:** multifidus *Spinal pain; segmental acupuncture*	D T1 to L1 M T1 to L5 S T1 to L5
Bladder line – Outer	3 *cun* lateral to the midline, on a vertical line joining the medial edge of the scapula and the outer border of the lumbar erector spinae **Angulation:** oblique towards spine **Target:** iliocostalis thoracis *Dorsal back pain, ventral pain* **CAUTION – do not needle deeply unless confident of angulation relative to pleura**	D T5 to T9 M T6 to T12 S T6 to T12 – rib level
BL44	Level with the lower border of T5	
BL45	Level with the lower border of T6	
BL46	Level with the lower border of T7	
BL47	Level with the lower border of T9	
BL48	Level with the lower border of T10	
BL49	Level with the lower border of T11	
BL50	Level with the lower border of T12	

FIGURE 16.10

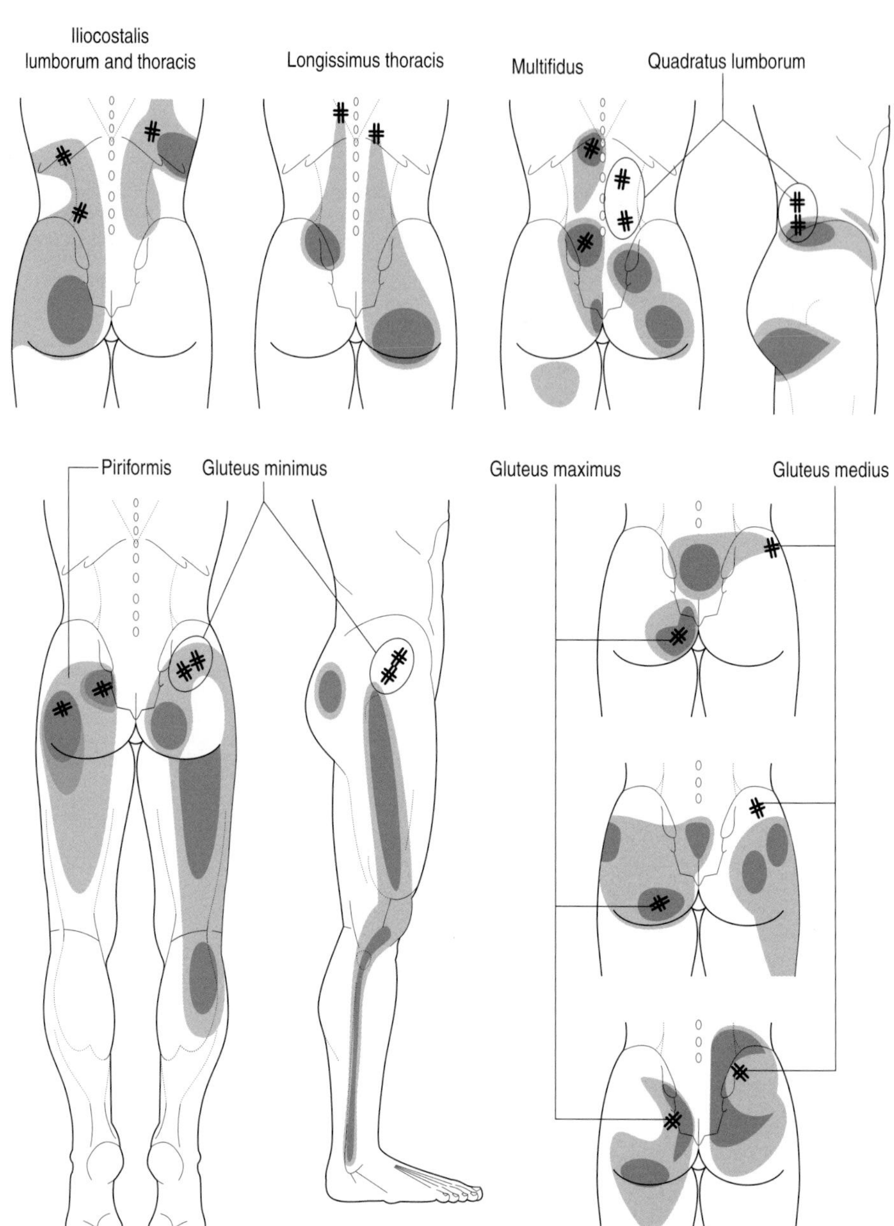

Figure 16.10 Low back and hip girdle: myofascial trigger points and pain reference zones.

FIGURE 16.11

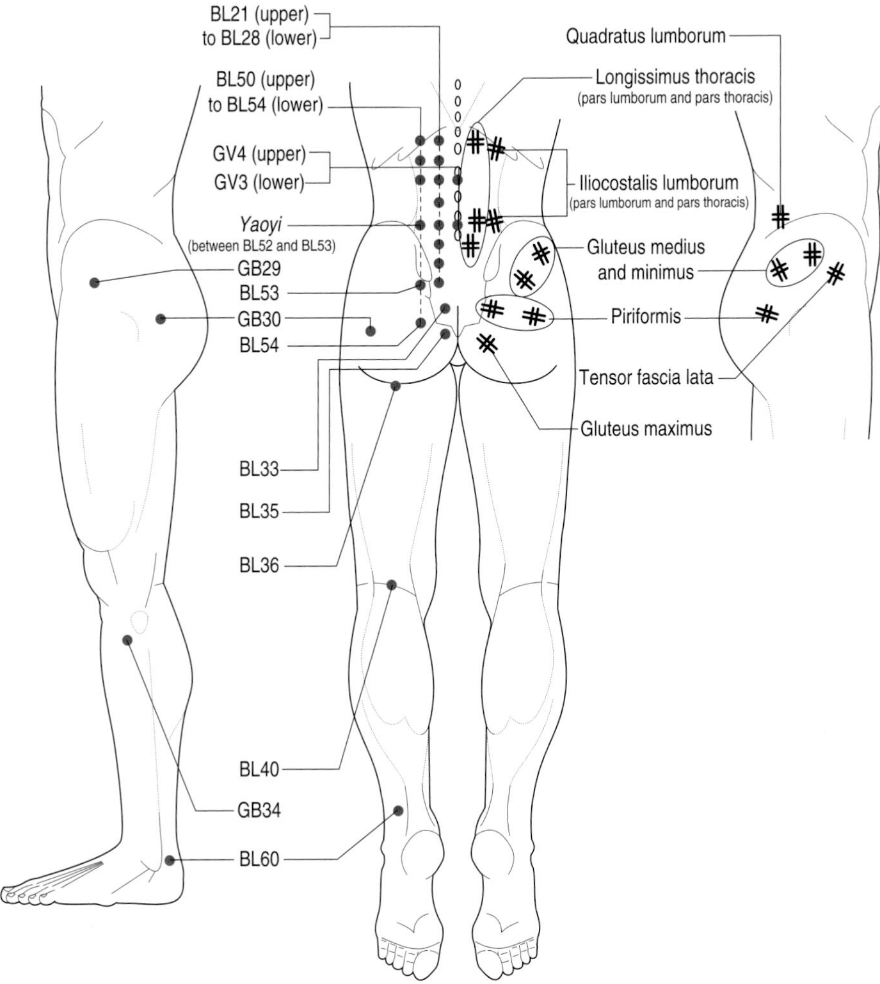

Figure 16.11 Low back and hip girdle: classical acupuncture points and trigger points.

TABLE 16.1.4

Table 16.1.4 Back and hip girdle

Lateral aspect		
GB29	Midway between the anterior superior iliac spine and the greater trochanter **Angulation:** perpendicular **Target:** tensor fasciae latae *Hip girdle pain* **CAUTION – deep needling may penetrate the capsule of the hip joint**	D L2/L3 M L5/S1/S2 S L4/L5/S1
GB30	1/3 of the way from the highest point of the greater trochanter to the sacral hiatus **Angulation:** towards symphysis pubis **Target:** tensor fasciae latae *Hip girdle pain, back pain, leg pain, sciatica* **CAUTION – avoid direct needling of the sciatic nerve**	D L2/L3 M L5/S1/S2 S L4/L5/S1
GB34	In the depression just anterior and inferior to the head of the fibula **Angulation:** perpendicular **Target:** peroneus longus *Leg pain; general point for musculoskeletal pain* **CAUTION – avoid needling the common fibular nerve**	D L5 M L5/S1 S L5
BL60	In the depression midway between the lateral malleolus and the Achilles tendon **Angulation:** perpendicular **Target:** connective tissue *Leg pain, Achilles tendon pain*	D L5/S1 M L5/S1 S S1/S2

Posterior aspect		
GV4	Between spinous processes L2 and L3 **Angulation:** transverse **Target:** interspinous ligament *Spinal pain*	D T9/T10 M L2 S L2
GV3	Between spinous processes L4 and L5 **Angulation:** transverse **Target:** interspinous ligament *Spinal pain*	D T11/T12 M L4 S L4
BL line – Inner	1.5 *cun* lateral to the midline, halfway between the Outer Bladder line and the spine **Angulation:** oblique towards spine **Target:** erector spinae *Back pain*	D T9 to S2 S T12 to S2
BL21	Level with the lower border of T12	M T10/T11
BL22	Level with the lower border of L1	M T11/T12
BL23	Level with the lower border of L2	M T12/L1
BL24	Level with the lower border of L3	M L1/L2
BL25	Level with the lower border of L4	M L2/L3
BL26	Level with the lower border of L5	M L3/L4

D = dermatome, M = myotome, S = sclerotome, n/a = not applicable
Meridian abbreviations – see Tables 16.6 and 16.7, page 218.

Posterior aspect		
BL27	Level with the S1 posterior foramen, or upper aspect of the posterior superior iliac spine **Angulation:** perpendicular **Target:** erector spinae or multifidus	M L4 S S1
BL28	Level with the S2 posterior foramen, or the lower aspect of the posterior superior iliac spine **Angulation:** perpendicular **Target:** erector spinae or multifidus	M L5 S S2
BL33	Over the S3 posterior foramen **Angulation:** perpendicular **Target:** S3 posterior foramen *Local pain; disturbance of pelvic organs, e.g. detrusor instability*	D S2/S3 M L5 S S3
BL35	0.5 *cun* lateral to the tip of the coccyx **Angulation:** perpendicular **Target:** sacrotuberous ligament *Coccydinia*	D S3/S4 M L5/S1/S2 S S4/ coccygeal
BL36	In the transverse gluteal crease, in a depression between the hamstring muscles **Angulation:** perpendicular **Target:** hamstring attachment *Local pain, hamstring pain, sciatica*	D S2/S3 M L5/S1/S2 S L5
BL40	On the popliteal crease midway between the tendons of biceps femoris and semitendinosus **Angulation:** perpendicular **Target:** connective tissue *Local pain, sciatica*	D S1/S2 M S1/S2 S n/a
BL line – Outer	3 *cun* lateral to the midline, on a vertical line joining the medial edge of the scapula and the outer border of the lumbar erector spinae **Angulation:** oblique towards spine unless stated otherwise below *Back pain*	D T9 to S2 S n/a mostly
BL50	Level with the lower border of T12	M T10/T11
BL51	Level with the lower border of L1	M T11/T12
BL52	Level with the lower border of L2	M T12/L1
Yaoyi	Level with the lower border of L4	M L2/L3
BL53	Level with the S2 posterior foramen, or the lower aspect of the posterior superior iliac spine **Angulation:** perpendicular **Target:** gluteus medius *Hip girdle pain, back pain*	D L2/S3 M L4 to S2 S L5
BL54	Level with the S4 posterior foramen in the sciatic notch **Angulation:** perpendicular **Target:** piriformis *Hip girdle pain, back pain, leg pain, sciatica* **CAUTION – avoid needling the sciatic nerve**	D S2/S3 M L5 to S2 S S2/S3
BL60	At the level of the most prominent part of the lateral malleolus, half way between it and the Achilles tendon **Angulation:** perpendicular **Target:** connective tissue space toward KI3 *Painful conditions, especially of spine, distant point in sciatica*	D L5/S1 M L5/S1 S n/a

FIGURE 16.12

Figure 16.12 Lower limb: myofascial trigger points and pain reference zones.

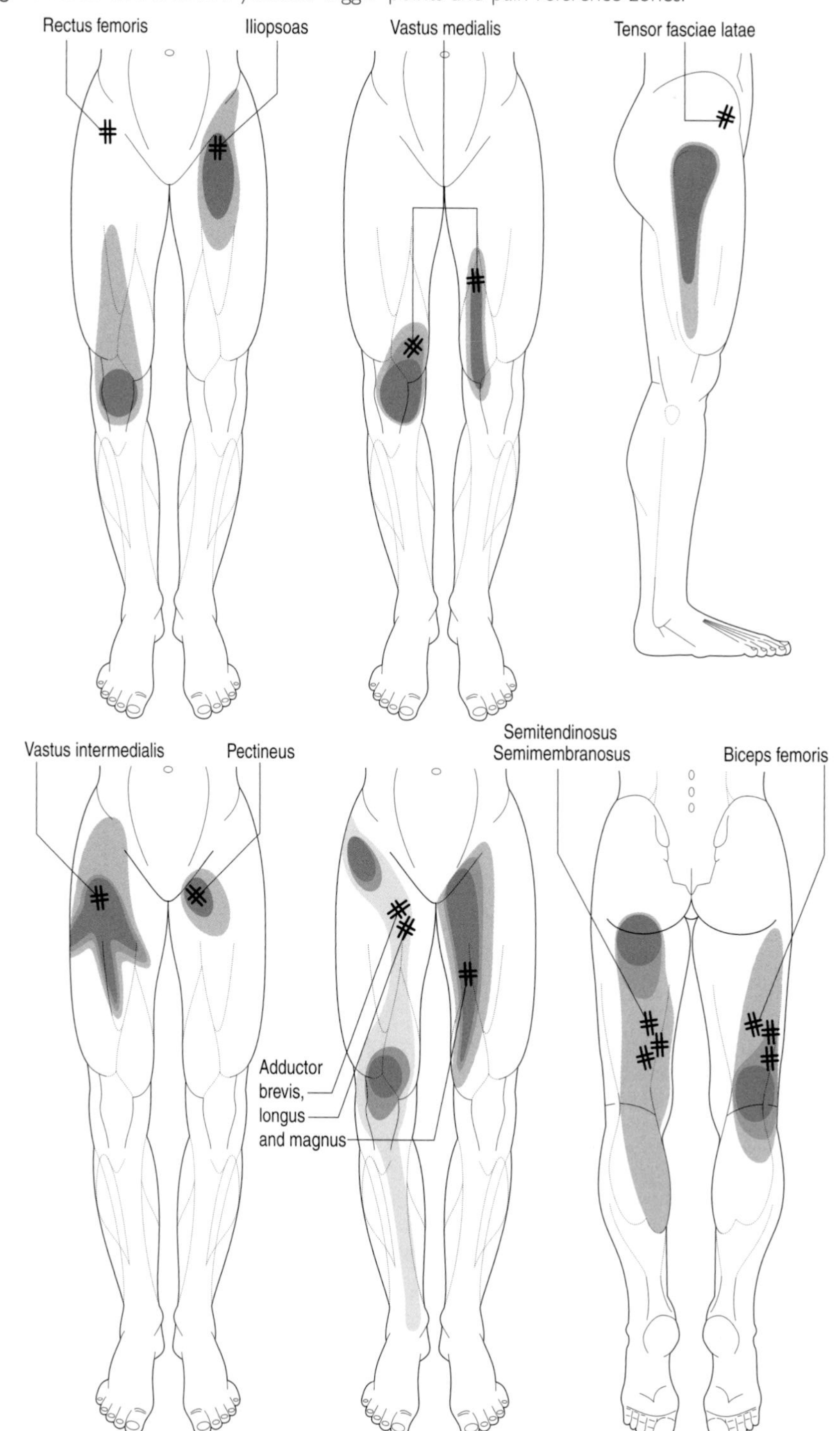

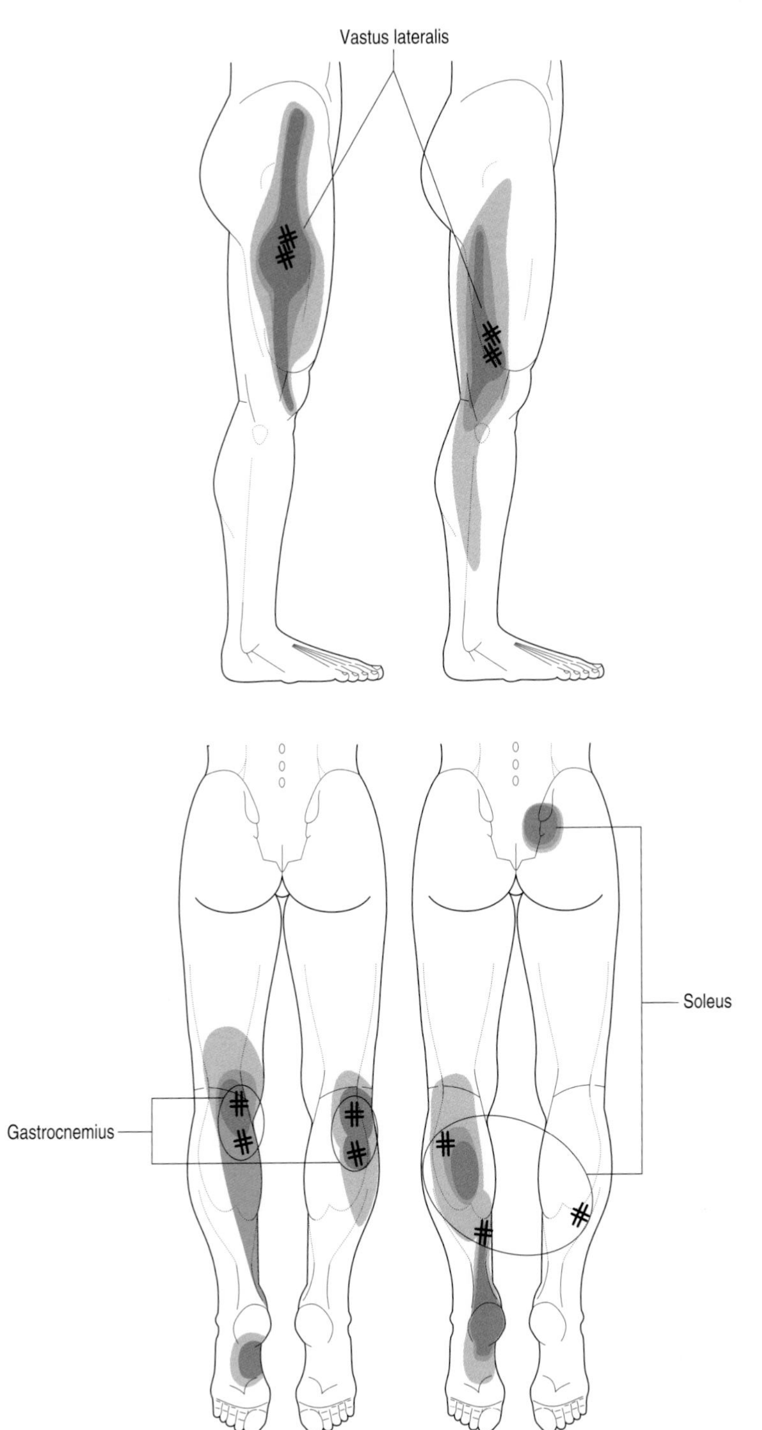
Vastus lateralis
Soleus
Gastrocnemius

FIGURE 16.13

Figure 16.13 Lower limb: classical acupuncture points and trigger points.

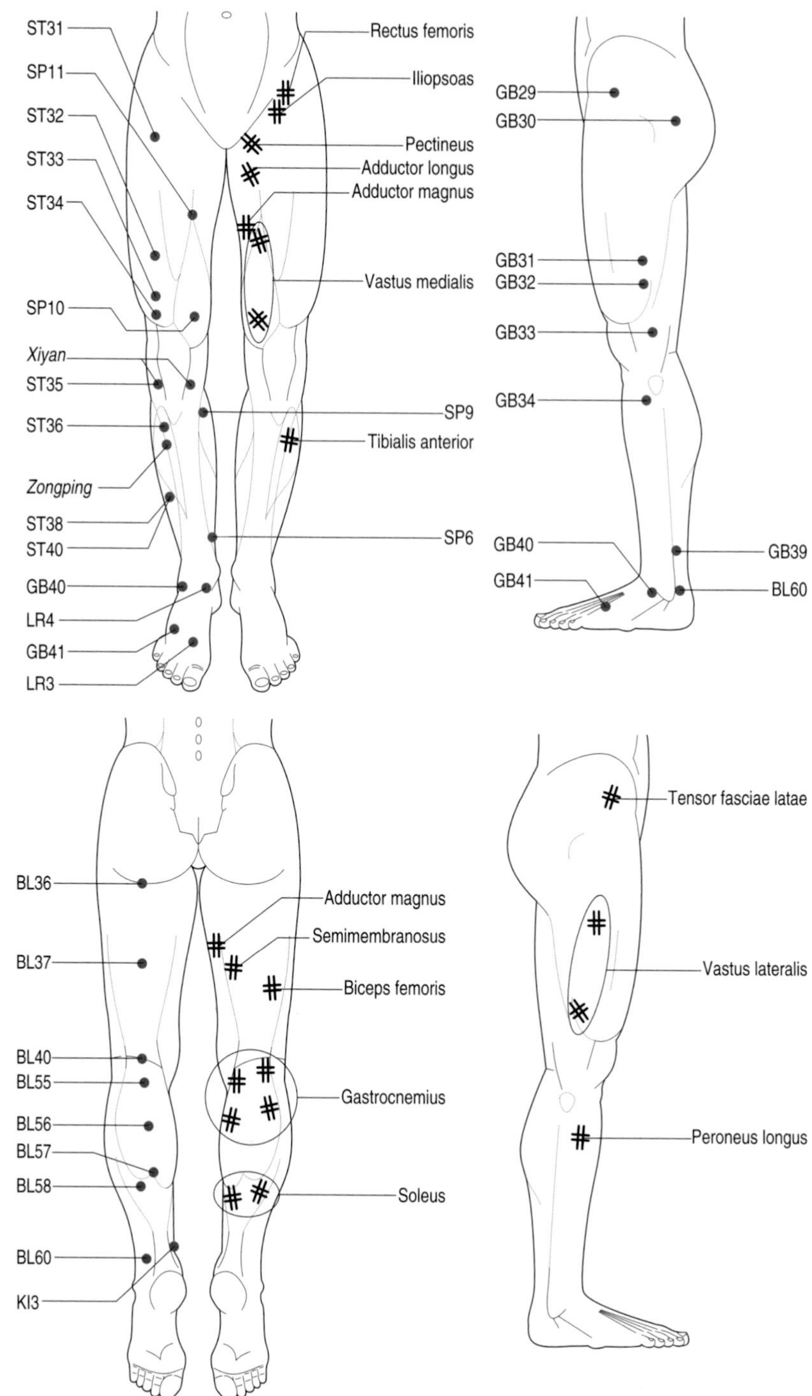

TABLE 16.1.5

Table 16.1.5 Lower limb

Thigh and lower leg: anterior aspect		
ST31	In a depression just lateral to sartorius, at the junction of a vertical line through the anterior superior iliac spine and a horizontal line at the level of the lower border of the pubic symphysis **Angulation:** perpendicular **Target:** rectus femoris *Thigh pain, anterior knee pain (rectus femoris)*	D L2 M L2/L3/L4 S L3/L4
ST32	6 *cun* superior to the upper lateral margin of the patella on a line that joins the lateral border of the patella to the anterior superior iliac spine **Angulation:** perpendicular **Target:** vastus lateralis *Thigh pain*	D L2 M L3/L4 S L3
ST33	3 *cun* superior to the upper lateral margin of the patella on a line that joins the lateral border of the patella to the anterior superior iliac spine **Angulation:** perpendicular **Target:** vastus lateralis *Thigh and knee pain*	D L2/L3 M L3/L4 S L3
ST34	2 *cun* superior to the upper lateral margin of the patella on a line that joins the lateral border of the patella to the anterior superior iliac spine **Angulation:** perpendicular **Target:** vastus lateralis *Knee pain*	D L2/L3 M L3/L4 S L3
ST35	In the hollow on the lateral aspect of the patella tendon directly over the joint line **Angulation:** towards the patella tendon [non-classical] **Target:** knee capsule *Knee pain* **CAUTION – avoid needling into the knee joint**	D L3/L4/L5 M L3/L4 S L3/L4/L5
Xiyan	In the hollows on either side of the patella tendon directly over the joint line **Angulation:** towards the patella tendon [non-classical] **Target:** knee capsule *Knee pain* **CAUTION – avoid needling into the knee joint**	D L3/L4/L5 M L3/L4 S L3/L4/L5
ST36	3 *cun* inferior to the knee joint, 1 fingerbreadth lateral to the lower border of the tibial tuberosity, in the middle of the upper third of the tibialis anterior **Angulation:** perpendicular **Target:** tibialis anterior *Knee pain, abdominal problems, major point for central effects*	D L4/L5 M L4/L5 S L4/L5
Zongping	1 *cun* inferior to ST36 **Angulation:** perpendicular **Target:** tibialis anterior *Used with ST36 for EA – major combination for central effects*	D L4/L5 M L4/L5 S L4/L5
ST40	On the anterolateral aspect of the lower leg, midway between the tibiofemoral joint line and the lateral malleolus, 2 fingerbreadths lateral to the anterior crest of the tibia **Angulation:** perpendicular **Target:** extensor hallucis longus *Local pain; a variety of traditional indications* **CAUTION – avoid needling to the depth of the anterior tibial artery**	D L5 M L5/S1 S L5/S1

D = dermatome, M = myotome, S = sclerotome, n/a = not applicable

Meridian abbreviations – see Tables 16.6 and 16.7, page 218.

continued

TABLE 16.1.5 continued

Table 16.1.5 Lower limb

Thigh and lower leg: anterior aspect		
SP11	6 *cun* superior to SP10, on a line connecting SP10 with SP12 **Angulation:** perpendicular **Target:** vastus medialis *Thigh and knee pain (vastus medialis)* **CAUTION – note the position of the femoral artery**	D L3 M L2/L3/L4 S L3
SP10	2 *cun* proximal to the superiomedial border of the patella, in the centre of vastus medialis **Angulation:** perpendicular **Target:** vastus medialis *Knee pain (vastus medialis)*	D L3 M L2/L3/L4 S L3
SP9	In a depression inferior to the medial condyle of the tibia and posterior to the medial border of the tibia, at the same level as GB34 **Angulation:** perpendicular **Target:** connective tissue space *Knee pain, gynaecological and urological problems*	D L3 M L2/L3/L4 S L3
SP6	3 *cun* superior to the most prominent part of the medial malleolus, on the medial border of the tibia **Angulation:** perpendicular **Target:** flexor digitorum longus *Gynaecological problems; major point for central effects*	D L4/S1/S2 M S1/S2 S L4/L5
LR4	Anterior to the medial malleolus, in the depression just medial to the tendon of tibialis anterior **Angulation:** perpendicular **Target:** connective tissue space *Ankle pain* **CAUTION – avoid needling into the ankle joint**	D L4/L5 M L4/L5 S L4/L5
LR3	On the dorsum of the foot, in the 1st metatarsal space, in a depression distal to the junction of the bases of the 1st and 2nd metatarsals **Angulation:** perpendicular **Target:** 1st dorsal interosseous *Local pain; headache; abdominal problems; major point for central effects* **CAUTION – the dorsalis pedis artery is at the apex of the 1st metatarsal space**	D L4/L5 M S2/S3 S L5/S1

Thigh and lower leg: lateral aspect		
GB29	On the lateral aspect of the hip midway between the anterior superior iliac spine and the greater trochanter **Angulation:** perpendicular **Target:** tensor fasciae latae or glutei *Hip girdle pain* **CAUTION – deep needling may penetrate the capsule of the hip joint**	D L2 M L4/L5/S1 S L3/L4/L5
GB30	1/3 of the way to the sacral hiatus from the most prominent part of the greater trochanter **Angulation:** perpendicular **Target:** lateral piriformis *Low back pain, hip girdle pain, sciatica* **CAUTION – avoid needling the sciatic nerve**	D L2/L3/S2 M L5/S1/S2 S L4/L5/S1
GB31	7 *cun* above the popliteal crease in the palpable furrow just posterior to the iliotibial tract **Angulation:** perpendicular **Target:** vastus lateralis or intermedius *Thigh and knee pain*	D L2 M L3/L4 S L3

D = dermatome, M = myotome, S = sclerotome, n/a = not applicable
Meridian abbreviations – see Tables 16.6 and 16.7, page 218.

Thigh and lower leg: lateral aspect

Point	Description	Innervation
GB32	In the palpable furrow just posterior to the iliotibial tract, 2 *cun* below GB32 **Angulation:** perpendicular **Target:** vastus lateralis or intermedius *Thigh and knee pain*	D L2 M L3/L4 S L3
GB33	On the lateral aspect of the knee 3 *cun* superior to GB34, in a depression between the femur and the tendon of biceps femoris **Angulation:** perpendicular **Target:** connective tissue space *Knee pain* **CAUTION – if the knee is flexed this point is close to the posterior joint margin**	D L2/L3/S2 M L4 to S2 S L3/L4
GB34	In the depression about 1 *cun* anterior and inferior to the head of the fibula **Angulation:** perpendicular **Target:** peroneus longus *Knee pain* **CAUTION – avoid deep needling since the anterior tibial artery and common fibular nerve are deep to this point**	D L5 M L5/S1 S L5
GB39	3 *cun* superior to the lateral malleolus, between the fibular shaft and the tendon of peroneus longus (use digital pressure to form a groove between the tendon and the fibula) **Angulation:** perpendicular **Target:** peroneus brevis *Lower leg and ankle pain* **CAUTION – avoid forceful ankle movement when a needle is placed in this point**	D L5/S1 M L5/S1 S L5/S1
GB40	In the depression anterior and inferior to the lateral malleolus **Angulation:** perpendicular **Target:** connective tissue space *Ankle pain* **CAUTION – avoid needling into the ankle joint**	D L5/S1 M L5/S1 S S1/S2
GB41	In the depression distal to the junction of the 4th and 5th metatarsals, lateral to the tendon of extensor digitorum longus that passes to the 5th toe **Angulation:** perpendicular **Target:** 4th dorsal interosseous *Forefoot pain*	D L5/S1 M S1/S2 S S2

continued

TABLE 16.1.5 continued

Table 16.1.5 Thigh and lower leg

Thigh and lower leg – posterior aspect		
BL36	In the transverse gluteal crease, in a depression between the hamstring muscles **Angulation:** perpendicular **Target:** hamstring attachment *Local pain, hamstring pain, sciatica*	D S2/S3 M L5/S1/S2 S L5
BL40	On the popliteal crease midway between the tendons of biceps femoris and semitendinosus, in the connective tissue space between the heads of gastrocnemius **Angulation:** perpendicular **Target:** connective tissue space *Local pain, sciatica* **CAUTION – note the popliteal artery and tibial nerve are deep to this point**	D S1/S2 M S1/S2 S n/a
BL55	2 *cun* inferior to BL40, on the line connecting BL40 and BL57, between the two heads of gastrocnemius **Angulation:** perpendicular **Target:** fascial plane *Calf pain*	D S1/S2 M S1/S2 S n/a
BL56	In the fascial plane between the heads of gastrocnemius, 5 *cun* below BL40, midway between BL55 and BL57 **Angulation:** perpendicular **Target:** fascial plane *Calf pain*	D S1/S2 M S1/S2 S n/a
BL57	In the depression formed below the bellies of the gastrocnemius muscle when the muscle is flexed, midway between BL40 and BL60 **Angulation:** perpendicular **Target:** musculotendinous junction *Calf pain*	D S1/S2 M S1/S2 S n/a
BL58	7 *cun* directly superior to BL60, lateral to and approximately 1 *cun* inferior to BL57, at the musculotendinous junction of the lateral head of gastrocnemius **Angulation:** perpendicular **Target:** musculotendinous junction *Calf pain*	D L5/S1/S2 M S1/S2 S n/a
BL60	At the level of the most prominent part of the lateral malleolus, half way between it and the Achilles tendon **Angulation:** perpendicular toward KI3 **Target:** connective tissue space *Painful conditions, especially of spine, distant point in sciatica*	D L5/S1 M L5/S1 S n/a
KI3	At the level of the most prominent part of the medial malleolus, half way between it and the Achilles tendon **Angulation:** perpendicular toward BL60 **Target:** connective tissue space *Ankle problems; urogenital problems; major point for central effects*	D L4/S2 M S2 S n/a

D = dermatome, M = myotome, S = sclerotome, n/a = not applicable
Meridian abbreviations – see Tables 16.6 and 16.7, page 218.

TABLE 16.2

Segmental levels of the autonomic innervation of the body

Part or organ of body	Sympathetic	Parasympathetic
Head and neck	T1 to T5	Four cranial nerves
Upper limb	T2 to T9	nil
Lower limb	T10 to L2	nil
Heart	T1 to T5	vagus
Lung and bronchi	T2 to T4	vagus
Oesophagus (caudal part)	T5 to T6	vagus
Stomach	T6 to T10	vagus
Small intestine	T9 to T10	vagus
Large intestine: to splenic flexure	T11 to L1	vagus
Large intestine: splenic flexure to rectum	L1 to L2	S2 to S4
Liver and gall bladder	T7 to T9	vagus
Testis and ovary	T10 to T11	nil
Urinary bladder	T11 to L2	S2 to S4
Uterus	T12 to L1	S2 to S4

TABLE 16.3

Spinal segmental levels and their relationship to acupuncture points

Region	Level	Dermatome	Myotome	Sclerotome[a]
Thoracic	1	GV14	LI4, SI3	
	2 to 8	see Figure 16.14	*Huatuojiaji* point at each level	
	9	GV4		
	10	GV4, BL23, ST25	ST25	
	11	BL23, BL25, GV3, CV4	CV4	
	12	BL25, GV3, CV4	BL23, CV4	
Lumbar	1		BL23	
	2		BL23, BL25, GV4, SP10	BL23, GV4
	3	SP9, L3	BL25, SP10	SP9
	4	ST36, SP6, SP9, KI3, LR3	BL25, ST36, SP10	BL25, ST36, SP6, SP9, KI3, GV3
	5	ST36, LR3	ST36, BL54(49)	ST36, LR3

continued

TABLE 16.3 continued

Spinal segmental levels and their relationship to acupuncture points continued

Region	Level	Dermatome	Myotome	Sclerotome[a]
Sacral	1	SP6, BL40(54)	SP6, SP9, KI3	LR3
	2	SP6, KI3, BL40(54)	SP6, SP9, KI3, LR3	KI3
	3	BL54(49)		
	4			
	5			

[a] Sclerotomal points include the spinous process at each vertebral level; and bony promontories near the classical point given in this table, e.g. for KI3, the medial malleolus.

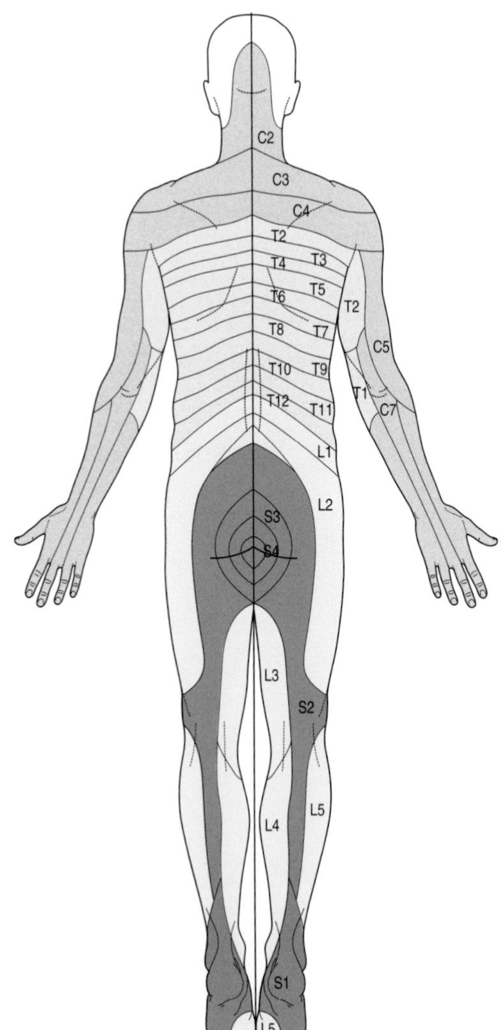

Figure 16.14 Dermatomes of the back (reproduced from Gray's Anatomy online, with permission of Elsevier).

TABLE 16.4

Innervation of some sites used for periosteal pecking

Target site for needling	Sclerotome
Occiput	C1
Acromion	C4
Spine of scapula	C4, C5
Greater tubercle of humerus	C5
Lateral epicondyle	C6, C7
Spinous process	Level of segment above (processes tend to angle inferiorly)
Iliac crest	L2
Greater trochanter	L5
Medial aspect of tibial plateau	L3, L4

TABLE 16.5

List of traditional points commonly regarded as 'major' points

Limb	Major points
Arm	LI11 LI4 TE5 PC6
Leg	ST36 SP6 LR3 KI3

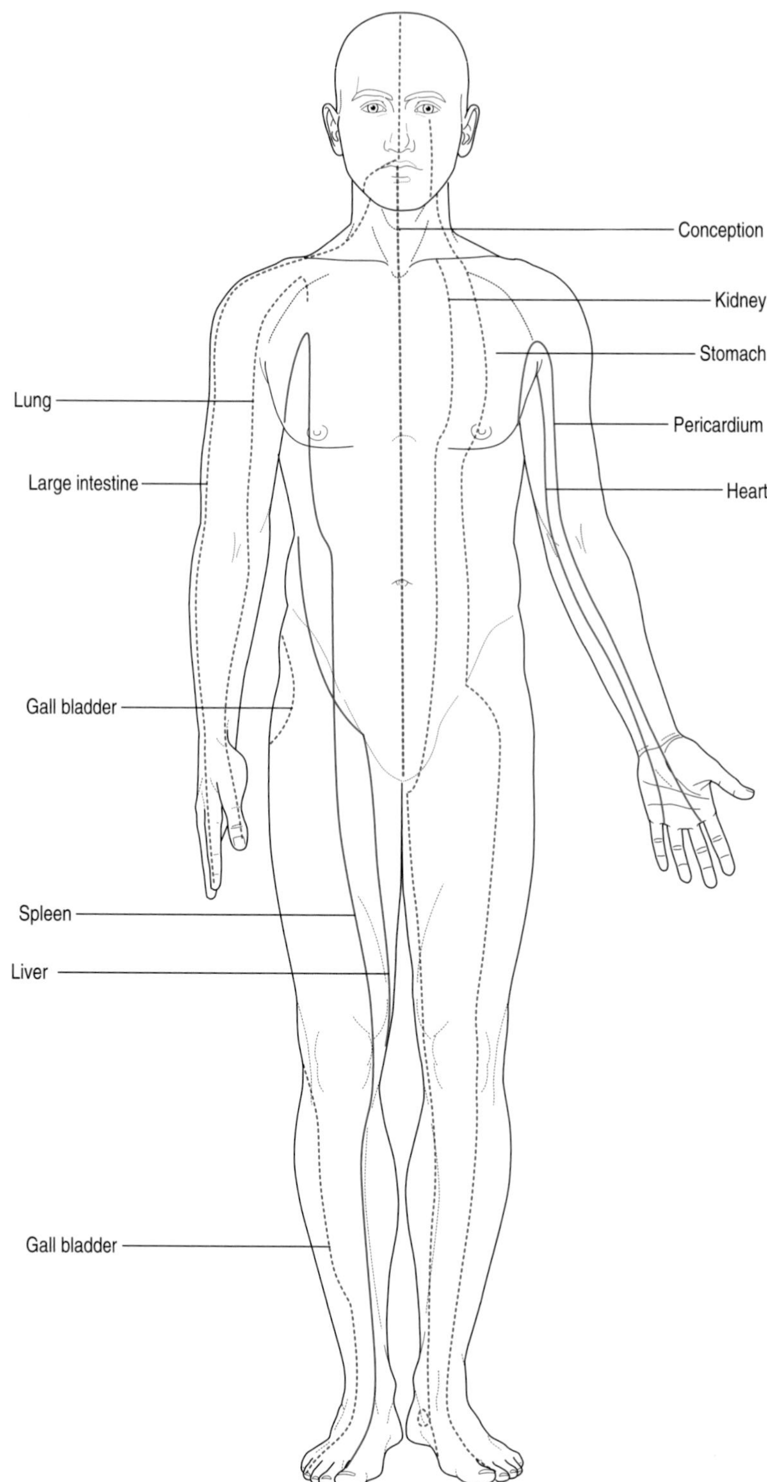

Figure 16.15 Anterior view of traditional meridians. Note that the Gall Bladder (GB) meridian is on the lateral surface and sections appear in each diagram.

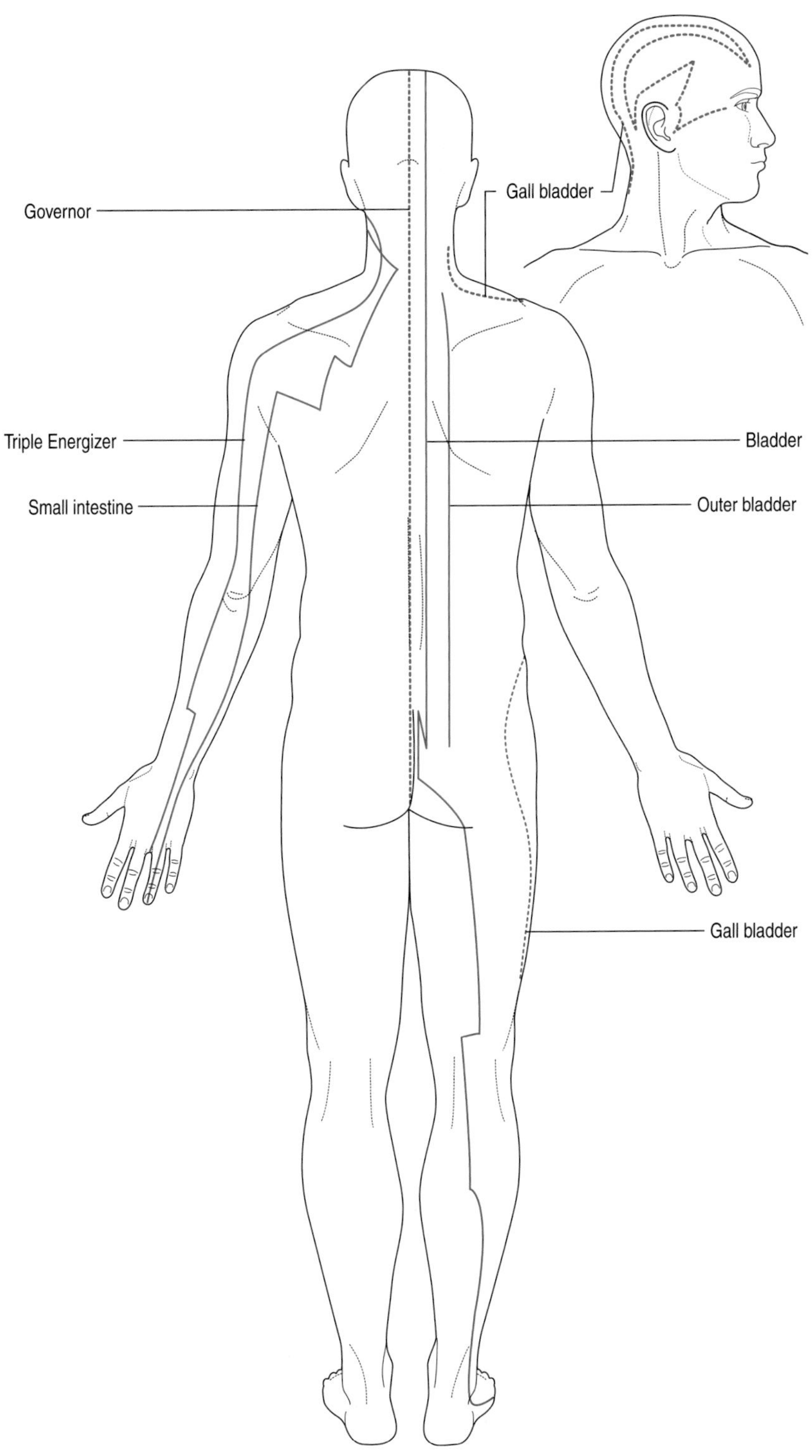

Figure 16.16 Posterior view of traditional meridians. Note that the Gall Bladder (GB) meridian is on the lateral surface and sections appear in each diagram.

TABLE 16.6

Meridians on the anterior surface of the body, their relevance to medical acupuncture, and alternative abbreviations

Meridian name and (abbreviation)	Significance of the meridian in medical acupuncture	Alternative abbreviations in other texts[a]
Lung (LU)	Little relevance	L, P
Pericardium (PC)	Relevant only in PC6	HC, Pe
Heart (HT)	Little relevance	C, He
Stomach (ST)	Useful on the abdomen and again around the knee	E, M
Spleen (SP)	Only relevant at points at the ankle and knee	LP, RP
Kidney (KI)	Little relevance, occasionally the abdomen points are useful	K, R, Rn
Liver (LR)	Relevant only at LR3	Liv, H, Lv
Conception vessel (CV)	Midline points that are relevant in both thorax and abdomen	Co, J, REN, VC

[a] Some abbreviations derive from names with Latin or French origin.

TABLE 16.7

Meridians on the posterior surface of the body, their relevance to medical acupuncture, and alternative abbreviations

Meridian name and (abbreviation)	Significance of the meridian in medical acupuncture	Alternative abbreviations in other texts[a]
Large Intestine (LI)	Points are used at hand, elbow and shoulder, and again at the final point near the nose	Co, IC
Triple Energizer (TE)	Relevant only in TE5	T, TB, TH, TW, SJ
Small Intestine (SI)	We meet this point at the medial border of the hand, and more points around the scapula	IT
Gall Bladder (GB)	Points are used around the neck and shoulder. Other points in the head, and in the leg, will also be useful	G, VB, VF
Bladder (BL)	A long meridian, and points are commonly used especially down the paraspinal region, and in the ankle	B, UB, VU
Governor vessel (GV)	Midline points are used in the lower and upper spine	DU, Go, TM, VG

[a] Some abbreviations derive from names with Latin or French origin.

REFERENCES

Allen J J B, Schnyer R N, Hitt S K 1998 The efficacy of acupuncture in the treatment of major depression in women. Psychological Science 9: 397–401

Alraek T, Baerheim A 2003 The effect of prophylactic acupuncture treatment in women with recurrent cystitis: kidney patients fare better. Journal of Alternative and Complementary Medicine 9(5): 651–658

Alraek T, Soedal L I, Fagerheim S U et al 2002 Acupuncture treatment in the prevention of uncomplicated recurrent lower urinary tract infections in adult women. American Journal of Public Health 92(10): 1609–1611

Andersson S, Lundeberg T 1995 Acupuncture – from empiricism to science: functional background to acupuncture effects in pain and disease. Medical Hypotheses 45(3): 271–281

Anon. 1823 Acupuncturation. Lancet November 9: 200–201

Baldry P E 1993 Acupuncture, trigger points and musculoskeletal pain. 2nd edn. Churchill Livingstone, Edinburgh

Baldry P 2005a The integration of acupuncture within medicine in the UK – the British Medical Acupuncture Society's 25th anniversary. Acupuncture in Medicine 23(1): 2–12

Baldry P E 2005b Acupuncture, trigger points and musculoskeletal pain. 3rd edn. Elsevier, Edinburgh

Basser S 1999 Acupuncture: a history. Scientific Review of Alternative Medicine 3(1): 34–41

Berman B, Ezzo J, Hadhazy V et al 1999 Is acupuncture effective in the treatment of fibromyalgia? Journal of Family Practice 48: 3–213

Birch S, Kaptchuk T 1999 History, nature and current practice of acupuncture: an East Asian perspective. In Ernst E, White A (eds) Acupuncture: a scientific appraisal. Butterworth-Heinemann, Oxford, pp 11–30

Bivens R E 2000 Acupuncture, expertise and cross-cultural medicine. Palgrave, Manchester

Blom M, Lundeberg T, Dawidson I et al 1993 Effects on local blood flux of acupuncture stimulation used to treat xerostomia in patients suffering from Sjögren's syndrome. Journal of Oral Rehabilitation 20: 541–548

Brattberg G 1986 Acupuncture treatments: a traffic hazard? American Journal of Acupuncture 14: 265–267

Bullock M L, Kiresuk T J, Sherman R E et al 2002 A large randomized placebo controlled study of auricular acupuncture for alcohol dependence. Journal of Substance Abuse Treatment 22(2): 71–77

Campbell A 2001 Acupuncture in practice: beyond points and meridians. Butterworth-Heinemann, Oxford

Carlsson C 2002 Acupuncture mechanisms for clinically relevant long-term effects – reconsideration and a hypothesis. Acupuncture in Medicine 20(2–3): 82–99

Ceccherelli F, Bordin M, Gagliardi G et al 2001 Comparison between superficial and deep acupuncture in the treatment of the shoulder's myofascial pain: a randomized and controlled study. Acupuncture and Electro-Therapeutics Research 26(4): 229–238

Chen Y 1997 Silk scrolls: earliest literature of meridian doctrine in ancient China. Acupuncture and Electro-Therapeutics Research 22: 175–189
Chiang C Y, Chang C T, Chu H L et al 1973 Peripheral afferent pathway for acupuncture analgesia. Scientia Sinica 16: 210
Chou C Y, Wen C Y, Kao M T et al 2005 Acupuncture in haemodialysis patients at the Quchi (LI11) acupoint for refractory uraemic pruritus. Nephrology Dialysis Transplantation 20(9): 1912–1915
Clement-Jones V, McLoughlin L, Tomlin S et al 1980 Increased beta-endorphin but not met-enkephalin levels in human cerebrospinal fluid after acupuncture for recurrent pain. Lancet 316: 945–947
Coyle M, Smith C 2005 A survey comparing TCM diagnosis, health status and medical diagnosis in women undergoing assisted reproduction. Acupuncture in Medicine 23(2): 62–69
Cummings T M 1996 A computerised audit of acupuncture in two populations: civilian and forces. Acupuncture in Medicine 14: 37–39
Cummings M, Lundeberg T 2006 Acupuncture for tinnitus. Complementary Therapies in Medicine 14(4): 290–291
Cummings T M, White A R 2001 Needling therapies in the management of myofascial trigger point pain: a systematic review. Archives of Physical Medicine and Rehabilitation 82(7): 986–992
Dawidson I, Angmar-Mansson B, Blom M et al 1998 The influence of sensory stimulation (acupuncture) on the release of neuropeptides in the saliva of healthy subjects. Life Sciences 63(8): 659–674
De Stefano R, Selvi E, Villanova M et al 2000 Image analysis quantification of substance P immunoreactivity in the trapezius muscle of patients with fibromyalgia and myofascial pain syndrome. Journal of Rheumatology 27(12): 2906–2910
Deluze C 1992 Electroacupuncture in fibromyalgia: results of a controlled trial. British Medical Journal 305(6864): 1249–1252
Diener H C, Kronfeld K, Boewing G et al 2006 Efficacy of acupuncture for the prophylaxis of migraine: a multicentre randomised controlled clinical trial. Lancet Neurology 5(4): 310–316
Dorfer L, Moser M, Bahr F et al 1999 A medical report from the stone age? Lancet 354: 1023–1025
Dorfer L, Moser M, Spindler K et al 1998 5200-year-old acupuncture in Central Europe? [letter]. Science 282: 242–243
Dyrehag L E, Widerstroem-Noga E G, Carlsson S G et al 1997 Effects of repeated sensory stimulation sessions (electro-acupuncture) on skin temperature in chronic pain patients. Scandinavian Journal of Rehabilitation Medicine 29: 243–250
Edwards J, Knowles N 2003 Superficial dry needling and active stretching in the treatment of myofascial pain – a randomised controlled trial. Acupuncture in Medicine 21(3): 80–86
Elden H, Ladfors L, Olsen M F et al 2005 Effects of acupuncture and stabilising exercises as adjunct to standard treatment in pregnant women with pelvic girdle pain: randomised single blind controlled trial. British Medical Journal 330(7494): 761–766
Ernst E, Pittler M H 1998 The effectiveness of acupuncture in treating acute dental pain: a systematic review. British Dental Journal: 443–447
Ernst G, Strzyz H, Hagmeister H 2003 Incidence of adverse effects during acupuncture therapy – a multicentre survey. Complementary Therapies in Medicine 11(2): 93–97
Ezzo J, Berman B, Hadhazy V et al 2000 Is acupuncture effective for the treatment of chronic pain? A systematic review. Pain 86(3): 217–225

Ezzo J, Vickers A, Richardson M A et al 2005 Acupuncture-point stimulation for chemotherapy-induced nausea and vomiting. Journal of Clinical Oncology 23(28): 7188–7198

Filshie J 2001 Safety aspects of acupuncture in palliative care. Acupuncture in Medicine 19(2): 117–122

Filshie J, Bolton T, Browne D et al 2005 Acupuncture and self acupuncture for long-term treatment of vasomotor symptoms in cancer patients – audit and treatment algorithm. Acupuncture in Medicine 23(4): 171–180

Filshie J, Hester J 2006 Guidelines for providing acupuncture treatment for cancer patients – a peer-reviewed sample policy document. Acupuncture in Medicine 24(4): 172–182

Filshie J, White A R 1998 Medical acupuncture: a Western scientific approach. Churchill Livingstone, Edinburgh

Fink M, Wolkenstein E, Karst M et al 2002 Acupuncture in chronic epicondylitis: a randomized controlled trial. Rheumatology (Oxford) 41(2): 205–209

Fujiwara H, Taniguchi K, Takeuchi J et al 1980 The influence of low frequency acupuncture on a demand pacemaker. Chest 78: 1285–1286

Fung K P, Chow O K W, So S Y 1986 Attenuation of exercise-induced asthma by acupuncture. Lancet 328: 1419–1422

Furlan A, Tulder M, Cherkin D et al 2005 Acupuncture and dry-needling for low back pain. Cochrane Database Systematic Reviews 1: CD001351

Gates S, Smith L, Foxcroft D 2006 Auricular acupuncture for cocaine dependence. Cochrane Database Systematic Reviews 1: CD005192

Gaudernack L C, Forbord S, Hole E 2006 Acupuncture administered after spontaneous rupture of membranes at term significantly reduces the length of birth and use of oxytocin. A randomized controlled trial. Acta Obstetricia et Gynecologica Scandinavica 85(11): 1348–1353

Gerwin R D, Shannon S, Hong C Z et al 1997 Interrater reliability in myofascial trigger point examination. Pain 69(1–2): 65–73

Haker E, Lundeberg T 1990 Acupuncture treatment in epicondylalgia: a comparative study of two acupuncture techniques. The Clinical Journal of Pain 6: 221–226

Han J S 2004 Acupuncture and endorphins. Neuroscience Letters 361(1–3): 258–261

Han J, Terenius L 1982 Neurochemical basis of acupuncture analgesia. Annual Review of Pharmacology and Toxicology 22: 193–220

Helms J M 1998 An overview of medical acupuncture. Alternative Therapies in Health and Medicine 4(3): 35–45

Hernandez-Diaz S, Rodriguez L A 2000 Association between nonsteroidal anti-inflammatory drugs and upper gastrointestinal tract bleeding/perforation: an overview of epidemiologic studies published in the 1990s. Archives of Internal Medicine 160(14): 2093–2099

Hoffman P 2001 Skin disinfection and acupuncture. Acupuncture in Medicine 19(2): 112–116

Hong C-Z 2000 Myofascial trigger points: pathophysiology and correlation with acupuncture points. Acupuncture in Medicine 18(1): 41–47

Hong C Z, Kuan T S, Chen J T et al 1997 Referred pain elicited by palpation and by needling of myofascial trigger points: a comparison. Archives of Physical Medicine and Rehabilitation 78(9): 957–960

Huang K C 1996 Side effects and mortality. Acupuncture: the past and the present. Vantage Press, New York, pp 251–254

Hubbard D R, Berkoff G M 1993 Myofascial trigger points show EMG activity. Spine 18: 1803–1807

Hughes J, Smith T W, Kosterlitz H W et al 1975 Identification of two related pentapeptides from the brain with potent opiate agonist activity. Nature 258(5536): 577–580

Hui K K, Liu J, Makris N et al 2000 Acupuncture modulates the limbic system and subcortical gray structures of the human brain: evidence from fMRI studies in normal subjects. Human Brain Mapping 9(1): 13–25

Hui K K S, Liu J, Marina O et al 2005 The integrated response of the human cerebro-cerebellar and limbic systems to acupuncture stimulation at ST 36 as evidenced by fMRI. Neuroimage 27(3): 479–496

Johansson B B 1993 Has sensory stimulation a role in stroke rehabilitation? Scandinavian Journal of Rehabilitation Medicine Suppl 29: 87–96

Kaplan G 1997 A brief history of acupuncture's journey to the West. Journal of Alternative and Complementary Medicine 3: S5–S10

Kaptchuk T 1983 Chinese medicine: the web that has no weaver. Rider, London

Karst M, Reinhard M, Thum P et al 2001 Needle acupuncture in tension-type headache: a randomized, placebo-controlled study. Cephalalgia 21(6): 637–642

Kelleher C J, Filshie J, Burton G et al 1994 Acupuncture and the treatment of irritative bladder symptoms. Acupuncture in Medicine 12(1): 9–12

Kellgren J H 1938 Observations on referred pain arising from muscle. Clinical Science 3: 175–190

Kendall D E 2002 Dao of Chinese medicine: understanding an ancient healing art. Oxford University Press, New York

Kleinhenz J, Streitberger K, Windeler J et al 1999 Randomised clinical trial comparing the effects of acupuncture and a newly designed placebo needle in rotator cuff tendinitis. Pain 83(2): 235–241

Knight B, Mudge C, Openshaw S et al 2001 Effect of acupuncture on nausea of pregnancy: a randomized, controlled trial. Obstetrics and Gynecology 97(2): 184–188

Lagrue G, Poupy J L, Grillot A et al 1977 Acupuncture anti-tabagique. La Nouvelle Presse Médicale 9: 966

Lao L, Bergman S, Anderson R et al 1994 The effect of acupuncture on post-operative pain. Acupuncture in Medicine 12: 13–17

Langevin H M, Bouffard N A, Badger G J et al 2006 Subcutaneous tissue fibroblast cytoskeletal remodeling induced by acupuncture: evidence for a mechanotransduction-based mechanism. Journal of Cell Physiology 207(3): 767–774

Lawson-Wood D, Lawson-Wood J 1973 The five elements of acupuncture and Chinese massage. Health Science Press, Holsworthy, Devon

Le Bars D, Dickenson A H, Besson J M 1979 Diffuse noxious inhibitory controls (DNIC). 1. Effects on dorsal horn convergent neurones in the rat. Pain 6: 283–304

Lee A, Copas J B, Henmi M et al 2006 Publication bias affected the estimate of postoperative nausea in an acupoint stimulation systematic review. Journal of Clinical Epidemiology 59(9): 980–983

Lee A, Done M 2004 Stimulation of the wrist acupuncture point P6 for preventing postoperative nausea and vomiting. Cochrane Database Systematic Reviews 3: CD003281

Lee H, Ernst E 2004 Acupuncture for labor pain management: A systematic review. American Journal of Obstetrics and Gynecology 191(5): 1573–1579

Lewith G T, Kenyon J N, Broomfield J et al 2001 Is electrodermal testing as effective as skin prick tests for diagnosing allergies? A double blind, randomised block design study. British Medical Journal 322(7279): 131–134

Lindall S 1999 Is acupuncture for pain relief in general practice cost-effective? Acupuncture in Medicine 17(2): 97–100

Linde K, Streng A, Hoppe A et al 2006 The programme for the evaluation of patient care with acupuncture (PEP-Ac) – a project sponsored by ten German social health insurance funds. Acupuncture in Medicine 24(Suppl): 25–32

Linde K, Streng A, Jurgens S et al 2005 Acupuncture for patients with migraine: a randomized controlled trial. Journal of the American Medical Association 293(17): 2118–2125

Lu G D, Needham J 1980 Celestial lancets: a history and rationale of acupuncture and moxa. Cambridge University Press, Cambridge

Lund I, Lundeberg T 2006 Are minimal, superficial or sham acupuncture procedures acceptable as inert placebo controls? Acupuncture in Medicine 24(1): 13–15

Lundeberg T 1999 Effects of sensory stimulation (acupuncture) on circulatory and immune systems. In Ernst E, White A (eds) Acupuncture: a scientific appraisal. Butterworth-Heinemann, Oxford

Ma K W 1992 The roots and development of Chinese acupuncture: from prehistory to early 20th century. Acupuncture in Medicine 10(Suppl): 92–99

MacDonald A J R 1982 Acupuncture: from ancient art to modern medicine. 1st edn. George Allen & Unwin, Boston

Maciocia G 1989 The foundations of Chinese medicine. Churchill Livingstone, Edinburgh

MacPherson H, Thomas K 2005 Short term reactions to acupuncture – a cross-sectional survey of patient reports. Acupuncture in Medicine 23(3): 112–120

MacPherson H, Thomas K, Walters S et al 2001 A prospective survey of adverse events and treatment reactions following 34,000 consultations with professional acupuncturists. Acupuncture in Medicine 19(2): 93–102

Manheimer E, White A, Berman B et al 2005 Meta-analysis: acupuncture for low back pain. Annals of Internal Medicine 142(8): 651–663

Manheimer E, Zhang G, Udoff L et al 2008 Effects of acupuncture on rates of pregnancy and live births among women undergoing in vitro fertilisation: systematic review and meta-analysis. British Medical Journal

Mann F 1992 Reinventing acupuncture. Butterworth-Heinemann, Oxford

Margolin A, Kleber H D, Avants S K et al 2002 Acupuncture for the treatment of cocaine addiction: a randomized controlled trial. Journal of the American Medical Association 287(1): 55–63

Martin D P, Sletten C D, Williams B A et al 2006 Improvement in fibromyalgia symptoms with acupuncture: results of a randomized controlled trial. Mayo Clinic Proceedings 81 (6): 749–757

Mayer D J, Price D D, Rafii A 1977 Antagonism of acupuncture analgesia in man by the narcotic antagonist naloxone. Brain Research 121: 368–372

McCarney R W, Brinkhaus B, Lasserson T J et al 2004 Acupuncture for chronic asthma. Cochrane Database Systematic Reviews 1: CD000008

Melchart D, Linde K, Fischer P et al 2001 Acupuncture for idiopathic headache (Cochrane Review). In: The Cochrane Library, Issue 3, 2001. Oxford: Update Publications 1: CD001218

Melchart D, Streng A, Hoppe A et al 2005 Acupuncture in patients with tension-type headache: randomised controlled trial. British Medical Journal 331(7513): 376–382

Melchart D, Thormaehlen J, Hager S et al 2003 Acupuncture versus placebo versus sumatriptan for early treatment of migraine attacks: a randomized controlled trial. Journal of Internal Medicine 253(2): 181–188

Melzack R, Stillwell D M, Fox E J 1977 Trigger points and acupuncture points for pain: correlations and implications. Pain 3: 3–23

Melzack R, Wall P D 1965 Pain mechanisms: a new theory. Science 150(699): 971–979

Melzack R, Wall P D 1988 The challenge of pain. Penguin Books, London

Mense S, Simons D G 1999 Muscle pain: understanding its nature, diagnosis and treatment. Lippincott Williams & Wilkins, Philadelphia

Myers C P 1991 Acupuncture in general practice: effect on drug expenditure. Acupuncture in Medicine 9: 71–72

Nesheim B I, Kinge R 2006 Performance of acupuncture as labor analgesia in the clinical setting. Acta Obstetricia et Gynecologica Scandinavica 85(4): 441–443

NIH Consensus Development Panel 1998 NIH Consensus Conference. Acupuncture. Journal of the American Medical Association 280(17): 1518–1524

Nogier P M F 1981 Handbook to Auriculotherapy. Maisonneuve, Moulin-les-Metz

O'Brien B, Relyea M J, Taerum T 1996 Efficacy of P6 acupressure in the treatment of nausea and vomiting during pregnancy. American Journal of Obstetrics and Gynecology 174: 708–715

Oomman S, Liu D, Cummings M 2005 Acupuncture for acute postoperative pain relief in a patient with pregnancy-induced thrombocytopenia – a case report. Acupuncture in Medicine 23(2): 83–85

Osler W 1912 The principles and practice of medicine. 8th edn. Appleton, New York

Pariente J, White P, Frackowiak R S et al 2005 Expectancy and belief modulate the neuronal substrates of pain treated by acupuncture. Neuroimage 25(4): 1161–1167

Park J, White A R, Ernst E 2000 Efficacy of acupuncture as a treatment for tinnitus: a systematic review. Archives of Otolaryngology – Head and Neck Surgery 126: 489–492

Peuker E, Cummings M 2003a Anatomy for the acupuncturist – facts & fiction 2: the chest, abdomen, and back. Acupuncture in Medicine 21(3): 72–79

Peuker E, Cummings M 2003b Anatomy for the acupuncturist – facts & fiction. 1: the head and neck region. Acupuncture in Medicine 21(1–2): 2–8

Peuker E, Cummings M 2003c Anatomy for the acupuncturist – facts & fiction. 3: upper & lower extremity. Acupuncture in Medicine 21(4): 122–132

Pomeranz B 2001 Acupuncture analgesia – basic research. In Stux G, Hammerschlag R (eds) Clinical acupuncture – scientific basis. Springer, Berlin

Pomeranz B, Chiu D 1976 Naloxone blockade of acupuncture analgesia: endorphin implicated. Life Sciences 19(11): 1757–1762

Ratcliffe J, Thomas K J, MacPherson H et al 2006 A randomised controlled trial of acupuncture care for persistent low back pain: cost effectiveness analysis. British Medical Journal 333(7569): 626–628A

Research Group of Acupuncture Anaesthesia 1974 The role of some neurotransmitters of brain in finger-acupuncture analgesia. Scientia Sinica 17: 112–130

Reston J 1971 Now about my operation in Peking. New York Times: 1,6

Ross J 2001 An audit of the impact of introducing microacupuncture into primary care. Acupuncture in Medicine 19(1): 43–45

Ross J, White A, Ernst E 1999 Western, minimal acupuncture for neck pain: a cohort study. Acupuncture in Medicine 17(1): 5–8

Sandberg M, Lundeberg T, Lindberg L G et al 2003 Effects of acupuncture on skin and muscle blood flow in healthy subjects. European Journal of Applied Physiology 90(1–2): 114–119

Sandkuhler J 2000 Learning and memory in pain pathways. Pain 88(2): 113–118

Scarsella S, Palattella A, Mariani P et al 1994 Electroacupuncture treatment of post-operative pain in oral surgery. Acupuncture in Medicine 12(2): 75–77

Scharf H P, Mansmann U, Streitberger K et al 2006 Acupuncture and knee osteoarthritis – a three-armed randomized trial. Annals of Internal Medicine 145(1): 12–20

Schnorrenberger C C 2003 Chen-Chiu: the original acupuncture, a new healing paradigm. Wisdom Publications, Somerville MA

Sciotti V M, Mittak V L, DiMarco L et al 2001 Clinical precision of myofascial trigger point location in the trapezius muscle. Pain 93(3): 259–266

Shah J P, Phillips T M, Danoff J V et al 2005 An in vivo microanalytical technique for measuring the local biochemical milieu of human skeletal muscle. Journal of Applied Physiology 99(5): 1977–1984

Simons D G, Travell J G, Simons L S 1999 Myofascial pain and dysfunction: the trigger point manual. Volume 1. Upper half of body. 2nd edn. Williams & Wilkins, Baltimore

Skootsky S A, Jaeger B, Oye R K 1989 Prevalence of myofascial pain in general internal medicine practice. Western Journal of Medicine 151(2): 157–160

Smith C, Crowther C, Beilby J 2002a Acupuncture to treat nausea and vomiting in early pregnancy: a randomized controlled trial. Birth 29(1): 1–9

Smith C, Crowther C, Beilby J 2002b Pregnancy outcome following women's participation in a randomised controlled trial of acupuncture to treat nausea and vomiting in early pregnancy. Complementary Therapies in Medicine 10(2): 78–83

Sola A E, Rodenberger M L, Gettys B B 1955 Incidence of hypersensitive areas in posterior shoulder muscles. American Journal of Physical Medicine 3: 585–590

Soulié de Morant G 1957 L'Acuponcture Chinoise. J. Lafitte, Paris

Stener-Victorin E, Humaidan P 2006 Use of acupuncture in female infertility and a summary of recent acupuncture studies related to embryo transfer. Acupuncture in Medicine 24(4): 157–163

Sze F K, Wong E, Yi X et al 2002 Does acupuncture have additional value to standard poststroke motor rehabilitation? Stroke 33(1): 186–194

The Academy of Traditional Chinese Medicine 1975 An outline of Chinese acupuncture. Foreign Languages Press, Peking

Thomas K J, MacPherson H, Ratcliffe J et al 2005 Longer term clinical and economic benefits of offering acupuncture care to patients with chronic low back pain. Health Technology Assessment Reports 9(32): 1–126

Thomas K J, Nicholl J P, Coleman P 2001a Use and expenditure on complementary medicine in England: a population based survey. Complement Therapies in Medicine 9(1): 2–11

Thomas K J, Nicholl J P, Fall M 2001b Access to complementary medicine via general practice. British Journal of General Practice 51(462): 25–30

Thomas M, Eriksson S V, Lundeberg T 1991 A comparative study of diazepam and acupuncture in patients with osteoarthritis. American Journal of Chinese Medicine 19: 95–100

Thomas M, Lundeberg T, Björk G et al 1995 Pain and discomfort in primary dysmenorrhoea is reduced by preemptive acupuncture or low frequency TENS. European Journal of Physical and Medical Rehabilitation 5(3): 71–76

Tough E A, White A R, Richards S et al 2007 Variability of criteria used to diagnose myofascial trigger point pain syndrome – evidence from a review of the literature. Clinical Journal of Pain 23(3): 278–286

Travell J G, Simons D G 1983 Myofascial pain and dysfunction: the trigger point manual. 1st edn. Williams & Wilkins, Baltimore

Travell J G, Simons D G 1992 Myofascial pain and dysfunction: the trigger point manual. Volume 2. The lower extremities. 1st edn. Williams & Wilkins, Baltimore

Trinh K, Graham N, Gross A et al 2007 Acupuncture for neck disorders. Spine 32(2): 236–243

Trinh K V, Phillips S D, Ho E et al 2004 Acupuncture for the alleviation of lateral epicondyle pain: a systematic review. Rheumatology (Oxford) 43(9): 1085–1090

Ulett G 1992 Beyond Yin and Yang: how acupuncture really works. Warren H Green, St Louis

Ulett G A, Han S-P 2002 The biology of acupuncture. Warren H Green, St Louis

Usichenko T I, Dinse M, Hermsen M et al 2005 Auricular acupuncture for pain relief after total hip arthroplasty – a randomized controlled study. Pain 114(3): 320–327

Uvnas-Moberg K, Bruzelius G, Alster P et al 1993 The antinociceptive effect of non-noxious sensory stimulation is mediated partly through oxytocinergic mechanisms. Acta Physiologica Scandinavica 149: 199–204

Veith I 1949 The yellow emperor's classic of internal medicine. University of California Press, Berkeley

Vickers A, Goyal N, Harland R et al 1998 Do certain countries produce only positive results? A systematic review of controlled trials. Controlled Clinical Trials 19(2): 159–166

Vickers A J, Rees R W, Zollman C E et al 2004 Acupuncture for chronic headache in primary care: large, pragmatic, randomised trial. British Medical Journal 328(7442): 744

Vincent C 2001 The safety of acupuncture. British Medical Journal 323(7311): 467–468

Vincent C A, Richardson P H, Black J J et al 1989 The significance of needle placement site in acupuncture. Journal of Psychosomatic Research 33: 489–496

Walsh B 2001 Control of infection in acupuncture. Acupuncture in Medicine 19(2): 109–111

Wang K, Yao S, Xian Y et al 1985 A study of the receptive field of acupoints and the relationship between the characteristics of needling sensation and groups of afferent fibres. Scientia Sinica 28: 963

Wedenberg K, Moen B, Norling A 2000 A prospective randomized study comparing acupuncture with physiotherapy for low-back and pelvic pain in pregnancy. Acta Obstetricia et Gynecologica Scandinavica 79(5): 331–335

White A 2004 A cumulative review of the range and incidence of significant adverse events associated with acupuncture. Acupuncture in Medicine 22(3): 122–133

White A 2006 The safety of acupuncture – evidence from the UK. Acupuncture in Medicine 24(Suppl): S53–S57

White A, Foster N E, Cummings M et al 2007 Acupuncture treatment for chronic knee pain: a systematic review. Rheumatology (Oxford) 46(3): 384–390

White A, Hayhoe S, Hart A et al 2001 Survey of adverse events following acupuncture (SAFA): a prospective study of 32,000 consultations. Acupuncture in Medicine 19(2): 84–92

White A, Kawakita K 2006 The evidence on acupuncture for knee osteoarthritis – editorial summary on the implications for health policy. Acupuncture in Medicine 24(Suppl): S71–S76

White A, Moody R 2006 The effects of auricular acupuncture on smoking cessation may not depend on the point chosen – an exploratory meta-analysis. Acupuncture in Medicine 24(4): 149–156

White A, Rampes H, Campbell J 2006 Acupuncture and related interventions for smoking cessation. Cochrane Database of Systematic Reviews 1: CD000009

White A R 2003 A review of controlled trials of acupuncture for women's reproductive health care. Journal of Family Planning and Reproductive Health Care 29(4): 233–236

White A R, Resch K L, Chan J C et al 2000 Acupuncture for episodic tension-type headache: a multicentre randomized controlled trial. Cephalalgia 20(7): 632–637

Witt C M, Brinkhaus B, Reinhold T et al 2006a Efficacy, effectiveness, safety and costs of acupuncture for chronic pain – results of a large research initiative. Acupuncture in Medicine 24(Suppl): S33–S39

Witt C M, Jena S, Brinkhaus B et al 2006b Acupuncture in patients with osteoarthritis of the knee or hip: a randomized, controlled trial with an additional nonrandomized arm. Arthritis and Rheumatism 54(11): 3485–3493

Witt C M, Jena S, Selim D et al 2006c Pragmatic randomized trial evaluating the clinical and economic effectiveness of acupuncture for chronic low back pain. American Journal of Epidemiology 164(5): 487–496

Wolfe F, Smythe H A, Yunus M B et al 1990 The American College of Rheumatology 1990 Criteria for the classification of fibromyalgia. Report of the Multicenter Criteria Committee. Arthritis and Rheumatism 33(2): 160–172

Wonderling D, Vickers A J, Grieve R et al 2004 Cost effectiveness analysis of a randomised trial of acupuncture for chronic headache in primary care. British Medical Journal 328(7442): 747–749

Woolf C J 1996 Windup and central sensitization are not equivalent. Pain 66(2–3): 105–108

Woollam C H M, Jackson A O 1998 Acupuncture in the management of chronic pain. Anaesthesia 53(6): 593–595

Wu M T, Hsieh J C, Xiong J et al 1999 Central nervous pathway for acupuncture stimulation: localization of processing with functional MR imaging of the brain – preliminary experience. Radiology 212(1): 133–141

Wu M T, Sheen J M, Chuang K H et al 2002 Neuronal specificity of acupuncture response: a fMRI study with electroacupuncture. Neuroimage 16(4): 1028–1037

Wyon Y, Lindgren R, Lundeberg T et al 1995 Effects of acupuncture on climacteric vasomotor symptoms, quality of life, and urinary excretion of neuropeptides among postmenopausal women. Menopause: the Journal of the North American Menopause Society 2: 3–12

Wyon Y, Wijma K, Nedstrand E et al 2004 A comparison of acupuncture and oral estradiol treatment of vasomotor symptoms in postmenopausal women. Climacteric 7(2): 153–164

Yamashita H, Tsukayama H, Hori N et al 2000 Incidence of adverse reactions associated with acupuncture. Journal of Alternative and Complementary Medicine 6: 345–350

Yamashita H, Tsukayama H, Tanno Y et al 1999 Adverse events in acupuncture and moxibustion treatment: a six-year survey at a national clinic in Japan. Journal of Alternative and Complementary Medicine 5(3): 229–236

Yoon SS, Kwon YK, Kim MR et al 2004 Acupuncture-mediated inhibition of ethanol-induced dopamine release in the rat nucleus accumbens through the GABA-B receptor. Neuroscience Letters 21; 369(3): 234–238

INDEX

Notes: Page numbers in *italics* refer to figures. Page numbers in **bold** refer to tables or boxed material. As the subject of this book is Western acupuncture, all entries refer to this type of acupuncture. The term 'traditional Chinese acupuncture' is used for classical treatment.

D

H

I

J

N

O

P

Q

R

S

Hartness Library
Vermont Technical College
One Main St.
Randolph Center, VT 05061
DISCARD